Workbook and Licensure Exam Prep for

RADIOGRAPHY ESSENTIALS

for Limited Practice

Third Edition

Workbook and Licensure Exam Prep for

RADIOGRAPHY ESSENTIALS
for Limited Practice

BRUCE W. LONG
MS, RT(R)(CV), FASRT
Director and Associate Professor
Radiologic Sciences Programs
Indiana University School of Medicine
Indianapolis, Indiana

EUGENE D. FRANK
MA, RT(R) FASRT, FAEIRS
Assistant Professor Emeritus
Mayo Clinic College of Medicine
Rochester, Minnesota

RUTH ANN EHRLICH
RT(R)
Retired, Radiology Faculty
Western States Chiropractic College
Portland, Oregon;
Adjunct Faculty
Portland Community College
Portland, Oregon

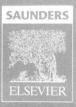

SAUNDERS

ELSEVIER

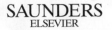

11830 Westline Industrial Drive
St. Louis, Missouri 63146

WORKBOOK AND LICENSURE EXAM PREP FOR
RADIOGRAPHY ESSENTIALS FOR LIMITED PRACTICE

ISBN: 978-1-4160-5765-9

Copyright © 2010, 2006, by Saunders, an imprint of Elsevier Inc.

Notice

Publisher: Jeanne Olson
Senior Developmental Editor: Linda Woodard
Publishing Services Manager: Catherine Jackson
Senior Project Manager: Gena Magouirk-Singh
Design Direction: Margaret Reid

Printed in the United States of America

Last digit is the print number: 9 8 7 6 5 4 3 2 1

Contents

Workbook and Licensure Exam Prep for

RADIOGRAPHY ESSENTIALS

for Limited Practice

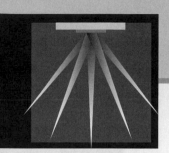

Learning Activities

Chapter 1

Role of the Limited X-ray Machine Operator

Exercise 1

Answer the following questions by selecting the best choice.

1. X-rays were discovered by:
   A. Eastman.
   B. Crookes.
   C. Edison.
   D. Roentgen.

2. The Joint Review Committee on Education in Radiologic Technology (JRCERT) is the:
   A. organization that accredits schools for radiologic technologists.
   B. organization that accredits schools for limited operators.
   C. professional organization for radiologic technologists.
   D. professional organization for limited operators.

3. Another term that has the same meaning as *practical radiographer* is:
   A. radiologic technologist.
   B. medical assistant.
   C. limited operator.
   D. imaging specialist.

4. (True/False) To determine the credentials needed for you to practice limited radiography, you should contact the appropriate state agency.

5. The term *limited* operator is used because the:
   A. scope of practice is limited.
   B. salaries are limited.
   C. opportunities are limited.
   D. radiographers' competence is limited.

6. *Reciprocity* means that:
   A. special credentials are required.
   B. credentials issued in one area are recognized in another.
   C. a license or permit has been applied for but has not been granted.
   D. there is freedom to practice without a license or permit.

7. Which of the following physicians has received extensive additional training and would be considered a specialist?
   1. Radiologist
   2. Obstetrician
   3. Pediatrician
   A. 1 and 2
   B. 1 and 3
   C. 2 and 3
   D. 1, 2, and 3

8. A specialist who interprets radiographs and performs special imaging procedures is called:
   A. a radiologic technologist.
   B. a chiropractor.
   C. a primary care physician.
   D. a radiologist.

9. An order for an x-ray examination is issued by:
   A. a physician.
   B. a nurse.
   C. a radiologic technologist.
   D. a medical assistant.

10. Which of the following are considered duties of a limited operator?
    1. Determine what examination should be performed
    2. Explain the procedure and the preparation to the patient
    3. Position the patient correctly in relation to the film and the x-ray tube
    A. 1 and 2
    B. 1 and 3
    C. 2 and 3
    D. 1, 2, and 3

11. The largest professional organization for radiologic technologists is the:
    A. ARRT.
    B. ASRT.
    C. JRCERT.
    D. ASSRT.

12. The curriculum for limited x-ray machine operators is published by the:
    A. ARRT.
    B. ASRT.
    C. JRCERT.
    D. ASSRT.

13. A podiatrist diagnoses and treats disorders and diseases of:
    A. the chest.
    B. the feet.
    C. children.
    D. the nervous system.

14. (True/False) Limited operators can perform the same x-ray examinations that radiographers can.

15. (True/False) Credentials for limited operators vary greatly from state to state.

Exercise 2

Answer the following questions.

1. When, where, and by whom were x-rays discovered?

   _____

   _____

2. What is the purpose of the ARRT? Why might this organization be important to a limited x-ray machine operator?

   _____

   _____

   _____

3. List possible consequences of practicing radiography outside the limitations imposed by local regulations.

   _____

   _____

   _____

   _____

4. What is the professional credential used by radiologic technologists after passing the ARRT examination in radiography and what does it stand for?

   _____

   _____

5. Explain what is meant by *reciprocity*.

   _____

   _____

6. List three activities that might take place in the "front office" of a clinic and four that typically occur in the "back office."

   Front office:

   1. _____

   2. _____

   3. _____

   Back office:

   1. _____

   2. _____

   3. _____

   4. _____

7. List five typical duties of a limited x-ray machine operator.

   1. _____

   2. _____

   3. _____

   4. _____

   5. _____

Exercise 3

Match the following terms with their definitions.

1. _____ Angiography

2. _____ Computed tomography

3. _____ Positron emission tomography

4. _____ Mammography

5. _____ Sonography

6. _____ Nuclear medicine

7. _____ Radiation therapy

8. _____ Magnetic resonance imaging

A. Treatment of malignant disease using radiation
B. Computerized imaging system that uses a powerful magnetic field and radiofrequency pulses to produce images of the body
C. Imaging of soft tissue structures using sound echoes
D. Imaging of blood vessels with the injection of special compounds called *contrast media*
E. Imaging of the breast using a special x-ray machine
F. Injection or ingestion of radioactive materials and the recording of their uptake in the body using a gamma camera
G. Computerized x-ray system that provides axial images (transverse "slices") of all parts of the body
H. A highly sophisticated computerized form of nuclear medical imaging

Exercise 4

Match the following health care specialties with their definitions.

1. _____ Anesthesiologist

2. _____ Geriatrician

3. _____ Obstetrician

4. _____ Oncologist

5. _____ Pediatrician

6. _____ Radiologist

7. _____ Orthopedist

8. _____ Thoracic specialist

A. Specializes in pregnancy, labor, delivery, and postpartum care
B. Specializes in problems and diseases of the elderly
C. Treats and diagnoses disorders and diseases in children
D. Specializes in diagnosis by means of medical imaging
E. Specializes in tumor identification and treatment
F. Administers anesthetics and monitors patients during surgery
G. Specializes in problems of the chest
H. Diagnoses and treats problems of the musculoskeletal system

Chapter 2

Introduction to Radiographic Equipment

Exercise I

Answer the following questions by selecting the best choice.

1. The x-ray room has an area that protects the limited operator from scatter radiation and is called the:
   A. control console.
   B. transformer.
   C. control booth.
   D. radiation field.

2. The mechanism on the x-ray tube crane that provides "stops" in a specific location is the:
   A. control console.
   B. transformer.
   C. tube port.
   D. detent.

3. The image that has been exposed on the film but has not been developed is called the:
   A. remnant radiation.
   B. scatter radiation.
   C. latent image.
   D. visible image.

4. The absorption of x-rays by matter is called:
   A. fog.
   B. attenuation.
   C. remnant radiation.
   D. exit radiation.

5. The image receptor (IR) system may consist of the following.
   A. Control console and transformer
   B. X-ray tube and tube stand
   C. Tube locks and detent
   D. Cassette and film

6. A line that is perpendicular to the long axis of the x-ray tube and is in the center of the x-ray beam is called the:
   A. central ray.
   B. scatter radiation.
   C. x-ray tube.
   D. primary x-ray beam.

7. The device that protects film from being fogged by scatter radiation is called a:
   A. detent.
   B. grid or Bucky.
   C. cassette.
   D. collimator.

8. The device that allows the limited operator to vary the size of the radiation field is called the:
   A. collimator.
   B. tube port.
   C. control console.
   D. detent.

9. The purpose of a safety check performed before making an exposure is to:
   A. ensure a quality radiographic image.
   B. prevent radiation hazard to oneself.
   C. prevent accidental exposure of co-workers.
   D. protect the patient from unnecessary exposure.

10. A radiation hazard exists in the x-ray room:
    A. throughout the room during an exposure.
    B. only in the path of the primary x-ray beam during an exposure.
    C. throughout the room at all times.
    D. throughout the room during exposure and for several minutes afterwards.

11. A type of filmless x-ray system that produces digital images is called:
    A. a remnant system.
    B. mobile radiography.
    C. an image receptor (IR).
    D. computed radiography (CR).

Exercise 2

Answer the following questions.

1. How can you determine the location of the central ray?

   _____

   _____

2. What is the location of remnant radiation?

   _____

   _____

3. What is meant by *attenuation?*

   _____

   _____

4. What component of the x-ray machine is located in the control booth?

   _____

   _____

5. What should you do before attempting to move the x-ray equipment?

   _____

   _____

6. Where would you look to find a collimator?

   _____

   _____

7. How might you determine the size of the radiation field without actually measuring it?

   _____

   _____

8. List the four steps in a preexposure safety check.

   1. _____

   2. _____

   3. _____

   4. _____

9. How soon is it safe to reenter the x-ray room after an exposure?

_____

_____

10. Define the difference between primary and remnant radiation.

_____

_____

_____

_____

11. Which common sizes of x-ray film are still manufactured in English dimensions?

_____

12. Describe the Trendelenburg position.

_____

_____

13. Describe the latent image.

_____

_____

Exercise 3

Match the following terms with their descriptions.

1. _____ Tube housing

2. _____ Tube port

3. _____ X-ray tube

4. _____ Scattered radiation

5. _____ Radiation fog

6. _____ Computed radiography (CR)

7. _____ Image receptor (IR)

A. Source of the x-rays
B. Unwanted image exposure that is caused by scattered x-rays
C. Surrounds the x-ray tube and is lined with lead
D. Filmless x-ray system that uses a digital format to produce images
E. Receives the energy of the x-ray beam and forms the image of the body part
F. Opening where the x-rays exit the tube
G. The x-rays that strike the patient and travel in all directions, inside and outside the body

Chapter 3

Basic Mathematics for Limited Operators

Exercise 1

Match the following terms with their definitions.

1. _____ Sum

A. The number that is "left over" when the dividend cannot be evenly divided by the divisor

2. _____ Difference

B. The answer to a multiplication problem

3. _____ Product

C. Total, the answer to an addition problem

4. _____ Dividend

D. The number by which the dividend is divided

5. _____ Divisor

E. The answer to a division problem

6. _____ Quotient

F. The answer to a subtraction problem

7. _____ Remainder

G. In a division problem, the number that is divided

Exercise 2

Answer the following questions.

1. The lower number of a fraction is called the _____ .

2. The upper number of a fraction is called the _____ .

3. A mixed number consists of a _____ and a _____ .

4. To multiply a whole number by a fraction, multiply the whole number by the

   _____ and then divide the product by

   the _____ .

5. Calculate the value of the following fractions of whole numbers.

   A. $\frac{1}{10} \times 80$ _____

   B. $\frac{1}{10} \times 200$ _____

C. ²/₅ × 150   _____

D. ¼ × 300   _____

E. ⁷/₁₀ × 80   _____

6. Reduce the following fractions to lowest terms.

A. ⁴/₁₀   _____

B. ³/₁₂   _____

C. ⁶/₁₈   _____

D. ¹²/₂₀   _____

E. ⁸/₂₄   _____

F. ¹⁵/₂₅   _____

G. ⁶/₈   _____

7. In a decimal, numerals to the left of the decimal point represent _____.

8. The first place to the right of the decimal point represents _____, the second

place represents _____, and the third place represents _____.

9. (True/False) 0.7 = 0.700.

10. (True/False) 3.3 = 3.03.

11. Set up the problems and calculate the sums of the following decimals.

A. 21.7 + 5.39 = _____

B. 33.06 + 30.2 = _____

C. 14.911 + 208.7 = _____

D. 29.844 + 3.3 + 27.6 = _____

E. 285.2 + 46.91 + 11.402 = _____

12. Set up the problems and calculate the differences of the following decimals.

A. 335.65 – 46.23 = _____

B. 456.33 – 3.87 = _____

C. 39.8 – 6.323 = _____

D. 21 – 7.51 = _____

E. 19.042 – 4.12 = _____

13. How do you determine where to place the decimal point in a problem that involves multiplication of decimals?

_____

_____

14. Set up the problems and calculate the products in the following problems involving multiplication of decimals.

A. $29.5 \times 5 =$ _____

B. $17.6 \times 40 =$ _____

C. $341.225 \times 48.33 =$ _____

D. $0.2213 \times 82.7 =$ _____

E. $83.22 \times 906.1 =$ _____

15. Set up the problems and calculate the quotients in the following problems involving division of decimals.

    A. $34.5 \div 5 =$ _____

    B. $720.35 \div 10 =$ _____

    C. $29 \div 2.5 =$ _____

    D. $284.31 \div 4.05 =$ _____

    E. $609.56 \div 6.22 =$ _____

16. To convert a fraction to a decimal, divide the _____ by the _____.

17. Convert the following fractions and mixed numbers to decimals.

    A. ⅛   _____

    B. ⅜   _____

    C. ⅟₆₀   _____

    D. ²⁄₁₅   _____

    E. 1¼   _____

18. *(Circle the correct phrase.)* When rounding off a decimal, drop the excess numerals from (left to right/right to left).

19. When rounding off a decimal, if the last numeral dropped is _____ or greater, increase the final

    remaining numeral by one; if the last numeral dropped is _____ or less, no change is necessary.

20. Round off the following decimals to the number of decimal places indicated in parentheses.

    A. 1.66666 (2)   _____

    B. 0.74139 (4)   _____

    C. 0.2509 (2)   _____

    D. 3.2551 (3)   _____

    E. 10.4444 (2)   _____

21. Perform the indicated calculations in the following problems by first converting the fractions to decimals. If decimals in this exercise have four or more decimal places, round them off to three decimal places.

    A. ¼ + ⅟₂₀ + ⅔= _____

    B. ³⁄₁₀ + ⅕ + ½ = _____

    C. ¾ – ⅜ = _____

    D. ²⁄₁₅ × 200 = _____

    E. ⅗ ÷ ½ = _____

22. (True/False) When adding or subtracting two percentages, the percentages must be converted to decimals.

23. (True/False) When multiplying or dividing percentages, or when performing calculations involving percentages and whole numbers, the percentages must be converted to decimals.

24. Convert the following percentages to decimals.

    A. 20%   _____

    B. 71.3%   _____

    C. 85%   _____

D. 69% _____

E. 172% _____

F. 800% _____

25. Convert the following decimals to percentages.

    A. 0.33 _____

    B. 0.4 _____

    C. 0.06 _____

    D. 1.89 _____

    E. 2.3 _____

    F. 6.0 _____

26. Perform the following calculations involving percentages.

    A. 73% + 27% = _____

    B. 50% + 25% = _____

    C. 30% – 3% = _____

    D. 20% × 60% = _____

    E. 79% × 30% = _____

    F. 25% ÷ 10% = _____

    G. 48% ÷ 2% = _____

27. Calculate the values of the following percentages up to 2 decimal places.

    A. 30% of 27 = _____

    B. 95% of 320 = _____

    C. 50% of 31 = _____

    D. 170% of 60 = _____

    E. 200% of 20 = _____

28. Determine the following percentages. Express your answers to the nearest tenth of a percent.

  A. 11 = _____% of 64

  B. 71 = _____% of 90

  C. 50 = _____% of 300

  D. 40 = _____% of 200

  E. 70 = _____% of 35

29. Calculate the solutions to the following problems that involve increasing and decreasing numbers by a percentage.

   A. Increase 75 by 15%.

   B. Increase 30 by 100%.

   C. Increase 12 by 20%.

   D. Decrease 85 by 10%.

   E. Decrease 50 by 12%.

30. A declaration that two mathematical statements (groups of numbers, together with their operational signs or mathematical functions) are equal to each other is called a(n) _____.

31. (True/False) The same symbols for mathematical operations used in arithmetic are also used in algebra.

32. *(Circle the correct word.)* The slanted line between the x and the 3 in the equation $x/3 = 6$ means that x is (multiplied/ divided) by 3.

33. (True/False) When an equation consists of two fractions, you can eliminate the denominators from consideration by using cross multiplication.

34. 3:4 is an example of a _____.

35. 3:4::6:8 is an example of a _____.

36. Determine the value of x up to three decimal places in each of the following equations.

    A. $2x + 9 = 11 = 3$

    B. $16/x = 12 - 4$

    C. $x - 61 + 12$

    D. $45 = 4x - 15$

    E. $3x = 9/3$

    F. $64 = 8x$

    G. $25/x = 10/2$

H. $x/3 = 48/12$

I. $72/8 = 80/x$

J. $10/x = 4/6$

37. Write the expression that indicates four cubed. _____

38. Write the expression that indicates five to the fifth power. _____

39. Calculate the values of the following exponential numbers.

A. 3^2

B. 3^3

C. 2^4

D. 9^2

E. 40^2

40. Write the square roots of the following numbers.

    A. 9 _____

    B. 16 _____

    C. 25 _____

    D. 81 _____

    E. 144 _____

41. Match the metric prefixes with their meanings.

    1. _____ Kilo-
    2. _____ Nano-
    3. _____ Milli-
    4. _____ Deci-
    5. _____ Hecto-
    6. _____ Centi-
    7. _____ Micro-
    8. _____ Deka-

    A. 10
    B. 100
    C. 1000
    D. $\frac{1}{10}$ (.1)
    E. $\frac{1}{100}$ (.01)
    F. $\frac{1}{1000}$ (.001)
    G. $\frac{1}{1,000,000}$ (.000001)
    H. $\frac{1}{1,000,000,000}$ (.0000000001)

42. Fill in the blanks in these statements of English measurement equivalents.

    A. One yard = _____ feet

    B. One foot = _____ inches

    C. One pint = _____ ounces

    D. One ton = _____ pounds

    E. One pound = _____ ounces

43. Fill in the blanks in these statements of metric equivalents.

    A. 1 meter = _____ centimeters

    B. 1 kilogram = _____ grams

    C. 1 liter = _____ milliliters

    D. 1 millisecond = _____ seconds

44. Convert the following metric measurements from one unit to another.

    A. Convert 70 kilovolts to volts.

    B. Convert 5 meters to centimeters.

    C. Convert 30 milliliters to liters.

    D. Convert 100 grams to kilograms.

    E. Convert 2 milligrams to grams.

45. Convert the following measurements from one English unit to another.

    A. Convert 18 inches to yards.

    B. Convert 2 quarts to fluid ounces.

    C. Convert 68 inches to feet.

    D. Convert 20 quarts to gallons.

    E. Convert 3.5 pounds to ounces.

46. Calculate the following conversions between English and metric units. Limit your answers to no more than four decimal places.

    A. Convert 5 fluid ounces to milliliters.

    B. Convert 100 pounds to kilograms.

    C. Convert 14 inches to meters.

    D. Convert 50 millimeters to inches.

    E. Convert 100 grams to ounces.

47. Calculate the following time and temperature conversions.

    A. Convert ⅟₆₀ second to milliseconds.

    B. Convert 260 seconds to hours.

    C. Convert 2.4 days to hours.

    D. Convert 75° F to the Celsius scale.

    E. Convert 25° C to the Fahrenheit scale.

48. Milliampere-seconds (mAs) is a useful unit in radiography because it indicates _____.

49. State the formula for determining mAs. _____.

50. When both mA and mAs are known, the formula for determining the exposure time is

    _____.

51. Calculate the mAs for the following exposures.

    A. 200 mA, 0.05 seconds

    B. 300 mA, 0.25 seconds

    C. 100 mA, 0.7 seconds

    D. 500 mA, $\frac{1}{20}$ seconds

    E. 50 mA, 0.3 seconds

    F. 150 mA, $1\frac{1}{4}$ seconds

    G. 400 mA, 2 milliseconds

52. Calculate the exposure time for the following exposures. Round any extended decimals to three decimal places.

    A. 50 mA, 10 mAs

    B. 200 mA, 40 mAs

C. 300 mA, 6 mAs

D. 100 mA, 2 mAs

E. 400 mA, 75 mAs

53. Write the formula for changing mAs to compensate for a change in source–image receptor distance (SID).

_____

54. Solve the following problems involving changes in SID.

A. What is the relative change in radiation intensity when the distance changes from 40 inches SID to 80 inches SID?

B. What is the relative change in radiation intensity when the distance is changed from 60 inches SID to 40 in SID?

C. A satisfactory radiograph is made using 25 mAs at 40 inches SID. How much mAs is needed to produce a similar radiograph at 48 inches SID?

D. A satisfactory radiograph is made using 30 mAs at 72 inches SID. How much mAs is needed to produce a similar radiograph at 84 inches SID?

E. A satisfactory radiograph is made using 12 mAs at 40 inches SID. How much mAs is needed to produce a similar radiograph at 72 inches SID?

55. Below 85 kVp, an adjustment of _____ kVp/cm will compensate for small changes in part size. Above 85 kVp, a change of _____ kVp/cm is necessary.

56. To compensate for a 2-cm *increase* in part size using mAs, increase the original mAs by _____%. To compensate for a 2-cm *decrease* in part size using mAs, decrease the original mAs by _____%.

57. Solve the following problems involving changes in patient part size.

   A. A satisfactory radiograph is made using 90 kVp on a patient part measuring 24 cm. Adjust the kVp to compensate for a patient part size decrease to 21 cm.

   B. A satisfactory radiograph is made using 72 kVp on a patient part measuring 16 cm. Adjust the kVp to compensate for a patient part size increase to 19 cm.

   C. A satisfactory radiograph is made using 20 mAs on a patient part measuring 22 cm. Adjust the mAs to compensate for a patient part size decrease to 20 cm.

   D. A satisfactory radiograph is made using 50 mAs on a patient part measuring 26 cm. Adjust the mAs to compensate for a patient part size increase to 30 cm.

   E. A satisfactory radiograph is made using 15 mAs on a patient part measuring 13 cm. Adjust the mAs to compensate for a patient part size increase to 15 cm.

58. *(Circle the correct word.)* The kVp is (increased/decreased) to shorten the scale of contrast.

59. *(Circle the correct word.)* When using the 15% rule to increase kVp, you must (multiply/divide) the mAs by 2.

60. Solve the following problems using the 15% rule.

   A. An exposure made using 20 mAs and 95 kVp has satisfactory radiographic density. Suggest a new technique that will provide more contrast.

   B. An exposure made using 120 mAs and 78 kVp has satisfactory radiographic density. Suggest a new technique that will decrease the patient dose.

   C. An exposure made using 20 mAs and 60 kVp has satisfactory radiographic density. Suggest a new technique that will provide more latitude.

   D. An exposure made using 25 mAs and 100 kVp has satisfactory radiographic density. Suggest a new technique that will provide more contrast.

   E. An exposure made using 30 mAs and 70 kVp has satisfactory radiographic density. Suggest a new technique that will provide less contrast.

61. *(Circle the correct word.)* The mAs is (directly/inversely) proportional to the relative speed of the image receptor system.

62. Use the grid conversion formula and the grid conversion factor table below to adjust mAs for the grid changes in the following problems.

Grid Conversion Factors

Grid Ratio	Grid Conversion Factor
No grid	1
5:1	2
8:1	4
12:1	5
16:1	6

A. If 30 mAs produces a satisfactory image using a 12:1 grid, state the mAs required with a grid ratio of 16:1.

B. If 4 mAs produces a satisfactory image without a grid, state the mAs required with a grid ratio of 8:1.

C. If 80 mAs produces a satisfactory image using a 12:1 grid, state the mAs required with a grid ratio of 8:1.

D. If 100 mAs produces a satisfactory image using a 16:1 grid, state the mAs required with a grid ratio of 12:1.

E. If 25 mAs produces a satisfactory image using a 12:1 grid, state the mAs required with no grid.

63. State the formula for determining the volume of medication that will deliver a specific dose.

64. Solve the following problems involving the calculation of medication quantities.

    A. The prescribed dose is 60 mg. The available stock is in the form of 15-mg tablets. How many should be given?

    B. The prescribed dose is 150 mg. The available stock has a strength of 50 mg/ml. How much should be given?

    C. The prescribed dose is 80 mcg. The available stock has a strength of 20 mcg/ml. How much should be given?

    D. The prescribed dose is 2 mg. The available stock has a strength of 1 mg/tablet. How much should be given?

    E. A toddler got into the medicine cabinet and ate four acetaminophen (Tylenol) tablets. The tablet strength is 500 mg. What dose did the child receive?

65. A physician prescribed a dose of 2 mg/kg of body weight for a child. The child weighs 40 lb. The drug is available in a strength of 4 mg/ml. How many milliliters should the child receive?

Chapter 4

Basic Physics for Radiography

Exercise 1

Answer the following questions by selecting the best choice.

1. Which of the following would be considered a basic form of matter?
   1. Solid
   2. Liquid
   3. Mass
   A. 1 and 2
   B. 1 and 3
   C. 2 and 3
   D. 1, 2, and 3

2. The quantity of matter that makes up any physical object is called the:
   A. nucleus.
   B. atomic number.
   C. mass.
   D. energy.

3. Which of the following is located in an orbit around the nucleus of an atom?
   A. Photon
   B. Electron
   C. Neutron
   D. Positron

4. Which of the following has a negative (–) electric charge?
   A. Neutron
   B. Proton
   C. Electron
   D. Positron

5. Which of the following are considered fundamental particles of atoms?
   1. Neutrons
   2. Photons
   3. Protons
   A. 1 and 2
   B. 1 and 3
   C. 2 and 3
   D. 1, 2, and 3

6. When a neutral atom gains or loses an electron, the atom is said to be:
   A. radioactive.
   B. unstable.
   C. ionized.
   D. neutral.

7. Mechanical energy can be classified as either kinetic energy or:
   A. magnetic energy.
   B. electromagnetic energy.
   C. chemical energy.
   D. potential energy.

8. X-rays consist of:
   A. electromagnetic energy.
   B. potential energy.
   C. chemical energy.
   D. thermal energy.

9. X-rays with greater energy have a shorter _____ and are more penetrating.
   A. frequency
   B. velocity
   C. wavelength
   D. potential difference

10. Of the following types of electromagnetic energy, which has the shortest wavelength?
    A. Radio waves
    B. Gamma rays
    C. Microwaves
    D. Ultraviolet light

11. Which of the following are accurate statements regarding the characteristics of x-rays?
    1. They are highly penetrating and invisible.
    2. They cause certain crystals to fluoresce.
    3. They travel in straight lines at the speed of light.
    A. 1 and 2
    B. 1 and 3
    C. 2 and 3
    D. 1, 2, and 3

12. The smallest possible unit of electromagnetic energy is the:
    A. photon.
    B. atom.
    C. nuclear energy.
    D. matter.

13. The term for a continuous path for the flow of electric charges from the power source through one or more electric devices and back to the source is:
    A. electric circuit.
    B. voltage.
    C. frequency.
    D. resistance.

14. The common unit of measure for the potential difference across an x-ray tube is the:
    A. ampere.
    B. milliampere.
    C. volt.
    D. kilovolt.

15. The frequency of alternating current delivered by electric utilities in the United States and Canada is:
    A. 120 V.
    B. 120 kV.
    C. 30 Hz.
    D. 60 Hz.

16. The purpose of a transformer is to:
    A. convert alternating current into direct current.
    B. convert direct current into alternating current.
    C. increase or decrease voltage.
    D. reduce the resistance in a circuit.

17. Which of the electron shells in the atom is most important for the production of x-rays?
    A. N
    B. M
    C. L
    D. K

18. (True/False) When a step-up transformer increases voltage from the primary to the secondary side of a transformer, amperage is increased.

19. (True/False) If a transformer has 100 turns on the primary side and 25 turns on the secondary side, it is a step-down transformer.

20. (True/False) A transformer with a 500:1 ratio would be a step-up transformer.

Exercise 2

Answer the following questions.

1. State the law of conservation of energy.

   _____

2. Name the electron orbit shell nearest the nucleus of an atom.

   _____

3. Name two forms of electromagnetic radiation that have a longer wavelength than diagnostic x-rays.

   1. _____

   2. _____

4. How does wavelength affect the usefulness of an x-ray beam?

   _____

   _____

5. What is meant by *ionization* and what determines the ionizing capability of electromagnetic radiation?

_____

_____

_____

_____

_____

6. List at least six characteristics of x-rays.

1. _____

2. _____

3. _____

4. _____

5. _____

6. _____

7. What is the velocity of x-rays? Are they faster or slower than visible light?

_____

_____

_____

_____

8. State the units used to measure current, potential difference, and electric resistance.

_____

_____

9. What does an ammeter measure? A voltmeter? How is each connected in a circuit?

_____

_____

_____

10. What is the duration of an electric cycle in the United States? An electric impulse?

_____

_____

_____

11. What is meant by electromagnetic induction?

_____

_____

12. What is the primary purpose of a transformer?

_____

_____

_____

Exercise 3

Match the following terms with their definitions.

1. _____ Ammeter

2. _____ Voltmeter

3. _____ Transformer

4. _____ Diode

5. _____ Kilovolt (kV)

6. _____ Ohm (Ω)

7. _____ Ampere (A)

8. _____ Milliampere (mA)

9. _____ Volt (V)

10. _____ Current

A. Quantity of electrons flowing in a circuit
B. Unit to measure the rate of current flow in a circuit
C. Equal to 1000 volts
D. Equal to 0.0001 A (¹⁄₁₀₀₀ A)
E. Allows electrons to flow in only one direction
F. Increases or decreases voltage by a fixed amount (alternating current only)
G. Measures electric current
H. Unit to measure resistance
I. Measures electric potential
J. Unit to measure potential difference

Chapter 5

X-ray Production

Exercise 1

Answer the following questions by selecting the best choice.

1. Roentgen discovered x-rays while working with a
   _____ tube.
   A. Coolidge
   B. Crookes
   C. Snook
   D. Edison

2. An "electron cloud" surrounding the filament of the
   cathode is referred to as a:
   A. space charge.
   B. photon.
   C. filament.
   D. focusing cup.

3. Free electrons for x-ray production come from the:
   A. filament.
   B. target.
   C. anode.
   D. focusing cup.

4. The creation of the space charge in the x-ray tube
   produces:
   A. resistance.
   B. variable resistance.
   C. conductivity.
   D. thermionic emission.

5. The majority of photons in the x-ray beam are
   created by which process?
   A. Characteristic interactions
   B. Bremsstrahlung interactions
   C. Magnetic induction
   D. Space charge

6. More than 99% of the energy of the electron stream
   is converted into:
   A. Bremsstrahlung photons.
   B. characteristic photons.
   C. secondary radiation.
   D. heat.

7. The high-speed rotation (10,000 rpm) of the anode
   enables:
   A. generation of a larger space charge.
   B. production of a greater number of electrons.
   C. greater dissipation of heat from high technical
      factors.
   D. focusing of the electron stream on a smaller area
      of the target.

8. The degree of angulation of the x-ray tube target
   will determine the:
   A. heat capacity of the tube.
   B. shape of the x-ray beam.
   C. size of the actual and effective focal spot.
   D. number of photons in the x-ray beam.

9. A dual-focus x-ray tube has:
   1. two filaments.
   2. two focal spot sizes.
   3. two focusing cups.
   A. 1 and 2
   B. 1 and 3
   C. 2 and 3
   D. 1, 2, and 3

10. The anode heel effect is a phenomenon of x-ray production that results in:
    A. dissipation of anode heat.
    B. uneven distribution of radiation within the x-ray field.
    C. filtration of the long x-ray wavelengths in the x-ray beam.
    D. production of characteristic radiation.

11. To take advantage of the anode heel effect when making a radiograph of the femur in recumbent anteroposterior projection on a 35 × 43 cm image receptor (IR) at a 40-inch source-image distance (SID), the patient should be placed so that the:
    A. head is toward the anode end of the tube.
    B. head is toward the cathode end of the tube.

12. The penetrating power of the x-ray beam is controlled by varying the:
    A. mA.
    B. kVp.
    C. anode speed.
    D. exposure time.

13. The rate of current flow across the x-ray tube is measured in:
    A. ohms.
    B. kilovolts.
    C. roentgens.
    D. milliamperes.

14. Doubling the mA will result in:
    1. increased patient dose.
    2. twice as many photons in the x-ray beam.
    3. increased radiographic density.
    A. 1 and 2
    B. 1 and 3
    C. 2 and 3
    D. 1, 2, and 3

15. The unit used to indicate the total quantity of x-ray exposure is:
    A. milliamperes.
    B. seconds (of exposure time).
    C. kilovolts.
    D. milliampere-seconds.

16. An x-ray exposure is made using the following factors: 200 mA, 0.02 seconds, 70 kVp, 40 inches SID. The value of the mAs for this exposure is:
    A. 0.04.
    B. 0.4.
    C. 4.
    D. 40.

17. The device for removing long-wavelength radiation from the primary x-ray beam is the:
    A. transformer.
    B. filter.
    C. rheostat.
    D. rectifier.

18. X-ray equipment capable or producing 70 kVp or more is required to have total filtration of at least:
    A. 0.5 mm aluminum equivalents (Al equiv).
    B. 1.5 mm Al equiv.
    C. 2.0 mm Al equiv.
    D. 2.5 mm Al equiv.

19. The purpose of rotating the anode of the x-ray tube is to:
    A. increase the heat capacity of the anode.
    B. increase the production of x-ray photons.
    C. decrease resistance in the circuit.
    D. decrease the size of the focal spot.

20. Image sharpness is determined by the:
    A. size of the electron stream.
    B. size of the actual focal spot.
    C. size of the effective focal spot.
    D. speed of rotation.

Exercise 2

Answer the following questions.

1. Describe the element tungsten. List two reasons why it is a good material for x-ray tube targets and at least one reason why it is used for x-ray tube filaments.

_____

_____

_____

Tube targets:

1. _____

2. _____

Tube filaments:

1. _____

2. What is meant by *thermionic emission*, and what is its purpose in the x-ray tube?

_____

_____

_____

3. What is meant by the term *heterogeneous* and what type of target interaction produces heterogeneous radiation?

_____

_____

_____

4. What does a dual-focus tube have that a single-focus tube does not?

_____

_____

_____

5. How much target angulation is needed in a general-purpose tube? Why?

_____

_____

_____

_____

6. What is the effect on the x-ray beam if the kVp is increased?

_____

_____

7. Why might it be desirable to increase mA? Why might it be undesirable?

_____

_____

_____

_____

8. An exposure is made using 100 mA and 0.25 sec. What is the value of the mAs? State another combination of mA and time that will produce the same quantity of exposure.

_____

_____

_____

9. If the x-ray tube has 0.5 mm Al equiv inherent filtration, and the collimator provides an additional 1.25 mm Al equiv, how much filtration must be added to meet minimum safety requirements?

_____

10. What is the standard rotation speed of the x-ray tube's anode?

_____

11. What is the percentage of characteristic radiation that is produced below 70 kVp?

_____

12. What is the difference in radiation intensity between the anode and cathode ends of the x-ray beam when a 35 × 43 cm IR is used at a 40-inch SID (state in percentage)?

_____

Exercise 3

Label the following drawings.

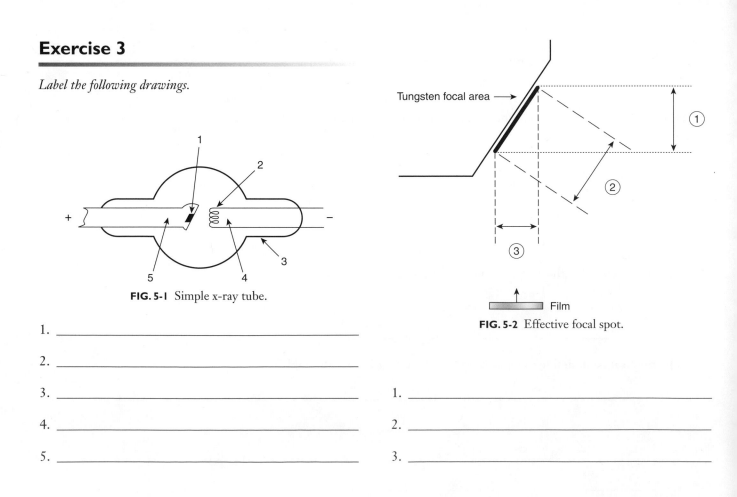

FIG. 5-1 Simple x-ray tube.

FIG. 5-2 Effective focal spot.

1. _____

2. _____

3. _____   1. _____

4. _____   2. _____

5. _____   3. _____

Exercise 4

Find the mAs for each of the technical factors below.

1.   20 mA × 1.00 sec = _____ mAs

2.   10 mA × 0.50 sec = _____ mAs

3. 100 mA × 0.75 sec = _____ mAs

4.   50 mA × 1.50 sec = _____ mAs

Determine the mA for each of the mAs values below.

5.   100 mAs = _____ mA × 2.00 sec

6.   200 mAs = _____ mA × 0.50 sec

7.   300 mAs = _____ mA × 1.50 sec

8.   75 mAs = _____ mA × 0.75 sec

Find the seconds for each of the mAs and mA values below.

9.   100 mAs = 100 mA × _____ sec

10.   200 mAs = 400 mA × _____ sec

11.   500 mAs = 250 mA × _____ sec

12.   300 mAs = 400 mA × _____ sec

Chapter 6

X-ray Circuit and Tube Heat Management

Exercise 1

Answer the following questions by selecting the best choice.

1. All of the following devices are located within the control console *except* the:
   A. step-up transformer.
   B. line meter.
   C. exposure switch.
   D. autotransformer.

2. A device that measures the voltage output from the autotransformer is the:
   A. kVp meter.
   B. line voltage meter.
   C. mA meter.
   D. exposure indicator.

3. The purpose of a line voltage compensator is to:
   A. select the kVp.
   B. select the mA.
   C. adjust the control for fluctuation in the electric supply.
   D. provide rectification of alternating current.

4. The mA selector is a device called a(n):
   A. line voltage meter.
   B. kVp meter.
   C. rheostat.
   D. exposure indicator.

5. A timer that is capable of producing ultrashort exposure times is typical of a(n):
   A. electronic timer.
   B. synchronous (impulse) timer.
   C. mechanical timer.
   D. phototimer.

6. The purpose of a rectifier in an x-ray circuit is to:
   A. vary the kVp.
   B. stabilize the kVp.
   C. measure current flowing.
   D. change alternating current (AC) into direct current (DC).

7. The following diagram represents the voltage waveform across an x-ray tube.

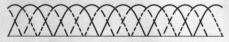

   FIG. 6-1 Voltage waveform across an x-ray tube.

   For this waveform, the x-ray machine has:
   A. self-rectification.
   B. rectified three-phase current.
   C. full-wave rectification.
   D. half-wave rectification.

8. The advantages of using a high-frequency generator instead of a single-phase generator include:
   1. reduction of patient dose.
   2. less exposure time to produce a given amount of exposure.
   3. a more constant voltage across the x-ray tube.
   A. 1 and 2
   B. 1 and 3
   C. 2 and 3
   D. 1, 2, and 3

9. How much can the exposure time be decreased when using three-phase x-ray equipment?
   A. 20%
   B. 30%
   C. 40% to 50%
   D. 50% to 60%

10. Automatic exposure control (AEC) automatically varies the:
    A. mA.
    B. kVp.
    C. exposure time.
    D. mA and kVp.

11. If the AEC fails during the exposure, the _____ will terminate the exposure.
    A. rectifier
    B. high-voltage circuit
    C. filament circuit
    D. back-up timer

12. According to the tube rating chart below, what is the maximum mAs obtainable at 90 kVp and 500 mA?

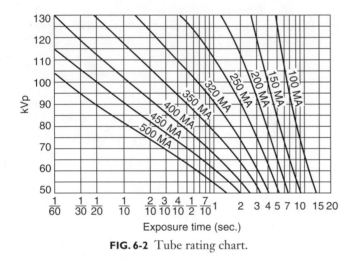

FIG. 6-2 Tube rating chart.

    A. 25 mAs
    B. 50 mAs
    C. 100 mAs
    D. 500 mAs

13. Which of the following steps should be used to extend x-ray tube life?
    1. Warm up the anode.
    2. Use high mA settings.
    3. Do not make repeated exposures near the tube limits.
    A. 1 and 2
    B. 1 and 3
    C. 2 and 3
    D. 1, 2, and 3

14. How many heat units (HU) are generated using a high-frequency generator at 200 mA, 0.10 sec, and 85 kVp?
    A. 1700 HU
    B. 2295 HU
    C. 2380 HU
    D. 3640 HU

15. For which type of x-ray generator can the exposure factors from the technique chart be programmed into the system?
    A. Manual exposure techniques
    B. Automatic exposure control (AEC)
    C. Anatomically programmed radiography (APR)
    D. Both B and C are correct.

16. For exposure times longer than 10 milliseconds, the maximum variability of the timer must be maintained within:
    A. ±3%
    B. ±5%
    C. ±10%
    D. ±4% to 6%

17. (True/False) Public Law 90-602 states that generators must terminate the exposure time at 400 mAs.

18. (True/False) When carrying out quality control of the kVp on the generator, the maximum variability has to be maintained within ±10%.

19. (True/False) The shortest exposure time and lowest dose to the patient is obtained using high-frequency generators.

20. (True/False) The heat unit (HU) formula for a three-phase x-ray generator is:

$$HU = mA \times Time \times kVp \times 1.35$$

Exercise 2

Label the following drawing.

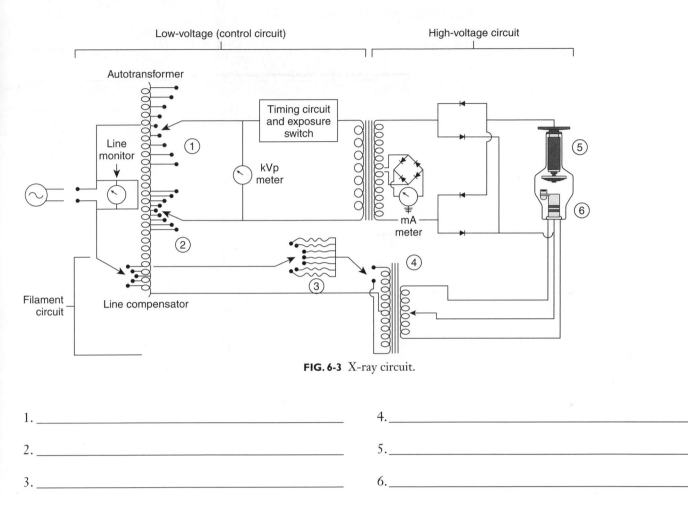

FIG. 6-3 X-ray circuit.

1. _____   4. _____

2. _____   5. _____

3. _____   6. _____

Exercise 3

Match the components listed below with one of the three following circuits.

　　1. Low-voltage circuit
　　2. Filament circuit
　　3. High-voltage circuit

A. _____ mA selector   G. _____ Autotransformer

B. _____ Rectifier unit   H. _____ Focal spot selector

C. _____ Line meter   I. _____ Line voltage compensator

D. _____ Rheostat   J. _____ Milliammeter

E. _____ X-ray tube   K. _____ kVp meter

F. _____ Step-down transformer   L. _____ Exposure timer

Exercise 4

Answer the following questions.

1. What causes fluctuations in line voltage? What should be done about it?

   _____

   _____

   _____

   _____

2. What is the primary purpose of the autotransformer?

   _____

   _____

   _____

3. What is the name of the device in the circuit that is represented on the control panel as the mA selector? Where in the x-ray circuit is it located?

   _____

   _____

4. What is the name of the device used to provide rectification in the x-ray circuit? How many are needed to provide full-wave rectification?

   _____

   _____

5. List two advantages of using a high-frequency x-ray generator compared with a single- or three-phase generator.

   1. _____

   2. _____

6. State, in order, the four steps for making an x-ray exposure after the control panel has been set.

   1. _____

   2. _____

   3. _____

   4. _____

7. Name two things that occur when the rotor switch is activated.

   1. _____

   2. _____

8. Name at least three features of an x-ray tube that are designed for handling the high heat.

   1. _____

   2. _____

   3. _____

9. For the tube rating chart shown on p. 42, what is the maximum amount of mAs that can be obtained at 80 kVp? What combination of mA and time will produce this amount of mAs?

   _____

   _____

10. If an exposure is made at 300 mA, 1 sec, and 90 kVp using a single-phase generator, how many heat units are generated at the anode?

    _____

11. Where is the center AEC detector located on a three-detector system?

    _____

12. The small focal spot is used when mA stations below _____ mA are used.

Chapter 7

Principles of Exposure and Image Quality

Exercise 1

Answer the following questions by selecting the best choice.

1. The unit used to indicate the total quantity of x-rays in an exposure is:
   A. mAs.
   B. seconds.
   C. kVp.
   D. mA.

2. Which of the following will result in increased radiographic density?
   1. Increased mA
   2. Increased exposure time
   3. Decreased source-image distance (SID)
   A. 1 and 2
   B. 1 and 3
   C. 2 and 3
   D. 1, 2, and 3

3. The mass density of the body part is referred to as:
   A. tissue density.
   B. radiographic density.
   C. radiographic contrast.
   D. subject contrast.

4. The primary controller of radiographic density is:
   A. SID.
   B. Object-image distance (OID).
   C. mAs.
   D. kVp.

5. The difference in radiographic density between any two adjacent portions of the image is called:
   A. tissue density.
   B. recorded detail.
   C. contrast.
   D. distortion.

6. The primary factor controlling radiographic contrast and x-ray penetration is:
   A. mA.
   B. exposure time.
   C. mAs.
   D. kVp.

7. High contrast produced by low kVp results in an image with:
   A. a long scale of contrast.
   B. a short scale of contrast.
   C. overpenetration.
   D. unsharpness.

8. Generalized unwanted exposure on the image is called:
   A. overexposure.
   B. overpenetration.
   C. fog.
   D. a long scale of contrast.

9. An decrease in SID will result in:
   A. increased magnification.
   B. underexposure.
   C. loss of contrast.
   D. decreased radiographic density.

10. A misrepresentation in the size or shape of the structure being examined is called:
    A. fog.
    B. distortion.
    C. unsharpness.
    D. recorded detail.

11. The "fuzzy" unsharpness at the edges of structures or body parts is called:
    A. fog.
    B. distortion.
    C. umbra.
    D. penumbra.

12. The smaller the effective focal spot, the _____ the penumbra, and the _____ the recorded detail.
    A. less, less
    B. less, greater
    C. greater, greater
    D. greater, less

13. When a large OID is used, recorded detail can be improved by:
    1. decreasing the SID.
    2. increasing the SID.
    3. maintaining the small focal spot.
    A. 1 and 2
    B. 1 and 3
    C. 2 and 3
    D. 1, 2, and 3

14. Fog affects radiographic quality by causing:
    A. decreased contrast.
    B. underexposure.
    C. increased contrast.
    D. distortion.

15. Motion of the patient, either voluntary or involuntary, during the exposure will result in decreased:
    A. contrast.
    B. distortion.
    C. radiographic density.
    D. detail.

16. A term used to describe a grainy or mottled image is:
    A. umbra.
    B. distortion.
    C. quantum mottle.
    D. penumbra.

17. Radiographic density is primarily controlled by adjusting the:
    A. SID.
    B. OID.
    C. mAs.
    D. kVp.

Exercise 2

Match the following terms with the corresponding definitions or descriptions.

1. _____ OID
2. _____ Penumbra
3. _____ Inverse square law
4. _____ SID
5. _____ Size distortion
6. _____ Elongation
7. _____ Shape distortion
8. _____ Foreshortening
9. _____ Density
10. _____ Long scale contrast
11. _____ Contrast
12. _____ Short scale contrast

A. Source–image receptor distance
B. Intensity is inversely proportional to the square of the distance
C. Object–image receptor distance
D. Result of unequal magnification
E. Overall blackness on the image
F. Magnification of a part
G. Unsharp edges
H. Difference in density between adjacent structures
I. Object appears shorter
J. Object appears longer
K. Produced by low kVp
L. Produced by high kVp

Exercise 3

Answer the following questions.

1. Which of the prime factors of exposure are directly proportional to the quantity of exposure?

   _____

2. What unit is used to indicate the total quantity of exposure?

   _____

3. If an exposure is made using 300 mA, 0.3 sec, 85 kVp, and 40 inches SID, what is the value of the mAs?

   _____

4. If the radiographic image is too dark, which exposure factor(s) would you change to solve the problem?

   _____

5. When it is desired to differentiate between tissues that have very similar tissue densities, is a long or short scale of contrast most desirable? Why?

   _____

   _____

6. What should you do if motion is anticipated in advance of making the exposure?

   _____

   _____

   _____

7. List two possible causes when a radiographic image appears gray and "flat."

   1. _____

   2. _____

8. If a large OID produces unacceptable loss of recorded detail, what other factors can be changed to improve the image?

   _____

   _____

9. When an overall radiographic image appears blurred, what aspect of image quality is affected? Which exposure factor might be changed to solve this problem?

   _____

   _____

10. List at least three measures that should be taken to prevent voluntary motion during radiography.

    1. _____

    2. _____

    3. _____

11. List at least three factors that will affect radiographic contrast.

    1. _____

    2. _____

    3. _____

12. List at least three factors that will affect distortion.

    1. _____

    2. _____

    3. _____

13. List at least four factors that will increase recorded detail in the radiographic image.

    1. _____

    2. _____

    3. _____

    4. _____

Chapter 8

Screen/Film Image Receptor Systems

Exercise I

Answer the following questions by selecting the best choice.

1. The function of a cassette is to:
   1. protect the film from exposure to light during use.
   2. protect the film from bending and scratching.
   3. increase the detail of the image.
   A. 1 and 2
   B. 1 and 3
   C. 2 and 3
   D. 1, 2, and 3

2. The purpose of intensifying screens is to:
   A. reduce the amount of exposure required to produce an image.
   B. increase the exposure needed to produce an image.
   C. increase the recorded detail of the image.
   D. increase the latitude of the exposure.

3. An intensifying screen with the smallest crystals will:
   1. require more mAs to maintain density.
   2. produce greater film density for a given amount of exposure.
   3. produce a radiographic image with more recorded detail.
   A. 1 and 2
   B. 1 and 3
   C. 2 and 3
   D. 1, 2, and 3

4. The phosphors commonly used for general-purpose intensifying screens today are:
   A. rare earth elements.
   B. calcium tungstate crystals.
   C. barium platinocyanoide.
   D. zinc sulfide.

5. An important rule to remember with respect to cleaning intensifying screens is:
   A. never pour liquid cleaner onto the screen.
   B. clean screens after every use.
   C. use a toothbrush to remove dust and dry dirt.
   D. when a liquid cleaner is needed, use mild soap and water.

6. Poor contact between the film and screen causes:
   A. lack of radiographic density.
   B. image blur.
   C. decreased screen speed.
   D. static artifacts.

7. Film emulsion consists of a mixture of gelatin and:
   A. rare earth phosphors.
   B. polyester.
   C. silver halide crystals.
   D. fluorides.

8. A wire mesh tool is used to test:
   A. screen speed.
   B. film/screen compatibility.
   C. spectral emission.
   D. film/screen contact.

9. The spectral sensitivity of the film must be matched to:
   A. the film speed.
   B. the screen speed.
   C. the color of light emitted by the screen.
   D. the processing chemicals.

10. The horizontal upper portion, or shoulder, of a sensitometric curve indicates:
    A. the radiographic density of a film base plus any accumulated fog.
    B. the maximum radiographic density produced by a film.
    C. the resolution of a film/screen combination.
    D. the compatibility of a film with an intensifying screen.

11. The use of intensifying screens reduces:
    1. exposure time.
    2. patient dose.
    3. mAs.
    A. 1 and 2
    B. 1 and 3
    C. 2 and 3
    D. 1, 2, and 3

12. Optimal film storage conditions include:
    1. a temperature of 50° to 70° F (10° to 21° C).
    2. protection from radiation exposure.
    3. 30% to 50% humidity.
    A. 1 and 2
    B. 1 and 3
    C. 2 and 3
    D. 1, 2, and 3

13. What percentage of the intensifying screen's light forms the x-ray image?
    A. 70%
    B. 99%
    C. 100%
    D. 70% to 99%

14. For general-purpose radiography, a relative screen speed (RS) of _____ is typically used.
    A. RS 100
    B. RS 200
    C. RS 300 to 400
    D. RS 400 to 600

15. As the screen speed increases, quantum mottle:
    A. increases.
    B. decreases.
    C. remains the same.
    D. can increase or decrease depending on the kVp.

16. A screen contact image should be viewed at a distance of at least:
    A. 3 feet.
    B. 4 feet.
    C. 5 feet.
    D. 9 feet.

Exercise 2

Fill in the blanks with T or F to indicate whether each of the following statements is true or false.

1. _____ Spectral emission refers to the color of light emitted by a phosphor.

2. _____ A radiopaque material is easily penetrated by the x-ray beam.

3. _____ The front of the cassette has a layer of lead foil that prevents backscatter.

4. _____ The ID blocker is for patient identification.

5. _____ A screen with greater efficiency requires less exposure and is said to be "faster."

6. _____ Screen speeds of RS 50 or RS 100 provide greater recorded detail.

7. _____ Damaged hinges on a cassette can cause poor film/screen contact.

8. _____ Inherent film characteristics may include sensitivity (speed), contrast, and spectral sensitivity.

9. _____ Films with larger crystals and thicker crystal layers produce a slower speed and greater detail.

10. _____ On the Hunter and Driffield curve (H & D curve), a steep, vertical curve indicates a long scale of contrast.

11. _____ A film with wide latitude will show more detail than a film with narrow latitude.

12. _____ The screen contact test should be performed quarterly.

Exercise 3

Answer the following questions.

1. What is the purpose of the lead foil layer in the cassette and where in the cassette is it located?

   _____

   _____

   _____

2. List three types of damage that may occur to a cassette and describe the problems created by each.

   1. _____

   2. _____

   3. _____

3. Compare the characteristics and performance of fast intensifying screens with slower or detail screens.

   _____

   _____

   _____

   _____

   _____

4. What colors are typical of the spectral emission of rare earth intensifying screens?

   _____

5. If you see a white image in the shape of a hair on a radiograph, what should you do?

   _____

   _____

   _____

   _____

6. What type of screen cleaning supplies should you keep in the radiology department?

   _____

   _____

   _____

   _____

7. Why is it a poor practice to stack x-ray film boxes flat on top of each other?

_____

_____

8. What is the optimum temperature for long-term x-ray film storage?

_____

9. State the film characteristic represented by each aspect of a sensitometric curve: toe, straight-line portion, straight-line slope, and shoulder.

_____

_____

_____

_____

10. Why is it important to match the spectral sensitivity of x-ray film to the spectral emission of the screen?

_____

_____

_____

_____

_____

11. What is the relative screen speed that is used for radiography of the limbs?

_____

12. Define the term *latitude*.

_____

_____

_____

Chapter 9

Digital Image Receptor Systems

Exercise 1

Match the following terms with their descriptions.

1. _____ Digital imaging

2. _____ Computed radiography

3. _____ Photostimulable phosphor plate

4. _____ Digital radiography

5. _____ Indirect conversion

6. _____ Direct conversion

7. _____ Postprocessing

A. A "cassette-less" digital x-ray system
B. A "cassette-based" digital x-ray system
C. Means for adjusting any image of a body part with computer software
D. Process in which detectors convert x-ray energy directly into an electric signal
E. General term for the process of acquiring images of the body using x-rays, displaying them digitally, and viewing and storing them on computers
F. Two-step process in which x-ray energy is converted to light and then to an electric signal
G. Stores the image of the body part

Exercise 2

Answer the following questions by selecting the best choice.

1. Which of the following modalities in radiology produce digital images that can be sent through a computer network?
   1. Computed tomography
   2. Magnetic resonance imaging
   3. Conventional radiography
   A. 1 and 2
   B. 1 and 3
   C. 2 and 3
   D. 1, 2, and 3

2. Which of the following is used in computed radiography (CR) to store a digital image?
   A. Laser light
   B. Photostimulable phosphor plate
   C. Flat panel detector
   D. Film/screen cassette

3. The phosphor used in the CR imaging plate is:
   A. lanthanum.
   B. gadolinium.
   C. yttrium.
   D. barium fluorohalide with europium.

4. Which of the following are necessary to process a CR radiographic image?
   1. Darkroom
   2. CR reader unit
   3. Computer systems with monitors
   A. 1 and 2
   B. 1 and 3
   C. 2 and 3
   D. 1, 2, and 3

5. After an imaging plate is scanned by the CR reader unit, it is erased with:
   A. laser light.
   B. white light.
   C. red light.
   D. fluorescent light.

6. One of the most important aspects of setting the exposure technique when using digital imaging systems is to ensure that which of the following is correctly set on the generator?
   A. kVp
   B. Source-image distance
   C. mA
   D. Exposure time

7. Which of the following is a true statement regarding the use of collimation with digital systems?
   A. At least two sides of collimation should be seen on the image.
   B. No collimation edges should be seen on the image.
   C. At least 1 cm of collimation should be seen on all four sides.
   D. At least 2 cm of collimation should be seen on two of the sides.

8. The erasure process will begin if a CR cassette is opened and the plate is exposed for:
   A. 5 seconds
   B. 10 seconds
   C. 15 seconds
   D. 20 seconds

Exercise 3

Fill in the blanks with the correct word or words.

1. With CR digital systems, the image plate is scanned with a _____ after being inserted into the reader device.

2. The phosphor plate inside the CR cassette can be used _____ times before it needs to be replaced.

3. The phosphor that absorbs the x-ray energy in a _____ system is called a *flat panel detector*.

4. Name at least two major advantages of using CR and digital radiography systems.

   1. _____

   2. _____

5. _____ will occur in digital systems if there are too few photons reaching the image receptor.

6. In digital radiography environments, the abbreviation *PACS* stands for

   _____.

7. _____ should be used for body parts that have extreme differences in tissue density.

8. Because of the wider dynamic range of digital systems, a *slightly* higher _____ setting may be acceptable for radiography projections done using a grid or Bucky.

9. If a CR plate is divided in half and used for two separate exposures, the side not receiving the exposure must

   always be _____.

10. The storage phosphors in CR plates are hypersensitive to _____.

Exercise 4

Fill in the blanks with T or F to indicate whether each of the following statements is true or false.

1. _____ An exposure technique chart is not necessary when using digital imaging systems.

2. _____ With direct conversion digital radiography, the x-ray energy is converted directly into an electric signal.

3. _____ Subtraction and contrast enhancement are postprocessing techniques.

4. _____ CR imaging plates should never be spit to enable two separate exposures on one plate.

5. _____ The image receptors used in digital radiography are much more sensitive to scatter radiation.

X-ray Darkroom and Film Processing

Exercise 1

Answer the following questions by selecting the best choice.

1. If a darkroom safelight test indicates that film may be fogged in the darkroom during routine handling, which of the following is a possible remedy for the problem?
   1. Replace the safelight bulb with a bulb of lower wattage.
   2. Check the darkroom for white light leaks.
   3. Check the safelight filter and replace if it is damaged or not the correct type.
   A. 1 and 2
   B. 1 and 3
   C. 2 and 3
   D. 1, 2, and 3

2. Sensitometers and densitometers should be calibrated:
   A. annually.
   B. semiannually.
   C. biennially.
   D. every 6 months.

3. Overreplenishment of processing chemicals in an automatic processor may result in:
   1. decreased radiographic density.
   2. decreased radiographic contrast and increased fog.
   3. incomplete drying of films.
   A. 1 and 2
   B. 1 and 3
   C. 2 and 3
   D. 1, 2, and 3

4. In a manual processing system, a 30-second rinse with agitation takes place upon completion of:
   A. washing.
   B. fixation.
   C. development.
   D. stop bath.

5. The operation of an automatic processor may include a:
   1. transport system.
   2. replenisher system.
   3. water system.
   A. 1 and 2
   B. 1 and 3
   C. 2 and 3
   D. 1, 2, and 3

6. Which of the following must be included in the monthly processor maintenance of a radiographic processor?
   1. Completely drain processing tanks.
   2. Measure cycle time with a stopwatch.
   3. Check developer temperature with a thermometer.
   A. 1 and 2
   B. 1 and 3
   C. 2 and 3
   D. 1, 2, and 3

7. The temperature for the developer solution in an automatic processing system is:
   A. 70° F (21.1° C).
   B. 75° F (23.9° C).
   C. 85° F (29.4° C).
   D. 95° F (35° C).

8. The Occupational Safety and Health Administration requires that personal protective equipment for chemical safety be used when:
   A. entering the darkroom.
   B. pouring processing chemicals or cleaning up chemical spills.
   C. processing radiographs in a manual processing system.
   D. processing radiographs in an automatic processor.

9. Which of the following equipment is necessary for monitoring processor performance?
    1. Sensitometer
    2. Densitometer
    3. pH meter
    A. 1 and 2
    B. 1 and 3
    C. 2 and 3
    D. 1, 2, and 3

10. A densitometer is a device used to:
    A. print a standard gray scale on film with a controlled light source.
    B. measure the transmission of light through an area of the film to determine the optical density.
    C. filter safelights to prevent darkroom fog.
    D. regulate replenishment in automatic processors.

11. Failure to agitate the film during manual development may result in artifacts on the radiograph that have the appearance of:
    A. pinholes.
    B. dark smudges.
    C. small, light circles.
    D. dark crescent marks.

12. An increase in the base + fog level on film may be caused by:
    1. use of outdated film.
    2. contamination of the film.
    3. safelight fog.
    A. 1 and 2
    B. 1 and 3
    C. 2 and 3
    D. 1, 2, and 3

13. The wash water tank of an automatic processor may be emptied at night to:
    A. decrease room humidity.
    B. prevent algae growth.
    C. prevent chemical odors.
    D. prevent contamination.

14. The type of filter used in the darkroom is a:
    A. No. 30.
    B. GBX.
    C. Wratten 3.
    D. Wratten 4.

15. How long should the film be exposed to the safelights when performing the darkroom safelight test?
    A. 2 minutes
    B. 3 minutes
    C. 4 minutes
    D. 5 minutes

16. At what density difference on the film from the darkroom safelight test should the safelight be adjusted or replaced?
    A. Greater than 0.05
    B. Greater than 0.06
    C. Less than 0.05
    D. Less than 0.06

17. How many 35 × 43 cm clean-out films should be run through the processor before any films are processed for the day?
    A. Two
    B. Three
    C. Four
    D. Five

18. When performing quality control procedures for the film processor, the speed index should be read at what density level on the control film?
    A. 1.00 above base + fog
    B. 1.25 above base + fog
    C. 1.50 above base + fog
    D. 2.00 above base + fog

Exercise 2

Label the following conditions as being caused by overreplenishment or underreplenishment of processing chemicals.

1. Loss of contrast _____

2. Loss of density _____

3. Inadequate hardening _____

4. Decreased maximum density _____

5. Inadequate clearing _____

6. Waste _____

Exercise 3

Answer the following questions.

1. What might cause you to suspect that a safelight was not safe? How would you find out whether it was safe? What would you do if it weren't?

_____

_____

_____

_____

_____

_____

_____

_____

2. What information must be included in the film identification?

_____

_____

_____

_____

3. State the primary function of the developer solution and two functions of the fixer solution.

Developer:

1. _____

Fixer:

1. _____

2. _____

4. How would you determine the minimum fixing time for a manual processing system?

_____

_____

_____

5. List three factors that would make it desirable to extend the wash time in a manual processing system beyond the usual 20 minutes.

   1. _____

   2. _____

   3. _____

6. Explain why replenisher solution for a manual developer needs to be stronger than the original solution. Why does fixer replenisher need to be stronger than the developer replenisher?

   _____

   _____

   _____

   _____

   _____

   _____

7. Two physicians from your clinic have gone on vacation, and you are now processing half as many films as usual in your automatic processor. This requires a change in replenishment rates. Should the rates be increased or decreased? How would you determine what the actual rates should be?

   _____

   _____

   _____

   _____

   _____

   _____

8. Your quality control film indicates an unacceptable increase in the base + fog index and a decrease in the contrast index. What are the possible causes? What can you do to identify the actual cause?

   _____

   _____

   _____

   _____

   _____

   _____

   _____

9. There has been an accidental spill of the used fixer holding container. What equipment will you need to clean it up? If you get some fixer in your eye, what should you do?

_____

_____

_____

_____

_____

Chapter 11

Scatter Radiation and Its Control

Exercise 1

Answer the following questions by selecting the best choice.

1. Radiation produced by the photoelectric effect is called:
   A. scattered radiation.
   B. Compton effect.
   C. secondary radiation.
   D. coherent scattering.

2. Scattered radiation affects the radiographic image by causing:
   1. fog.
   2. reduced contrast.
   3. reduced recorded detail.
   A. 1 and 2
   B. 1 and 3
   C. 2 and 3
   D. 1, 2, and 3

3. Which of the following factors will affect the quantity of scattered radiation fog on a radiograph?
   1. kVp
   2. Screen speed
   3. Field size
   A. 1 and 2
   B. 1 and 3
   C. 2 and 3
   D. 1, 2, and 3

4. The most effective method of reducing scattered radiation fog on a radiograph is to:
   A. decrease the object-image distance (OID).
   B. decrease the source-image distance (SID).
   C. increase the kVp.
   D. use a grid or Bucky.

5. The effectiveness of a grid is determined by the grid ratio, which is:
   A. the relationship between the height of the lead strips and the width of the spaces between them.
   B. the SID at which the grid is designed to be used.
   C. the number of lead strips per inch.
   D. the grid's focal range.

6. As compared with an 8:1 ratio grid, a 12:1 ratio grid will:
   A. clean up scattered radiation more effectively.
   B. require less precise centering.
   C. require less exposure to make a satisfactory radiograph.
   D. produce less radiographic contrast.

7. On a radiograph, the appearance of decreased density on the side of the image is most likely caused by:
   A. grid motion.
   B. grid cutoff.
   C. grid ratio.
   D. grid frequency.

8. A moving grid may be part of a radiographic table or upright unit and is called a:
   A. Bucky grid.
   B. crosshatch grid.
   C. focused grid.
   D. linear grid.

9. The frequency of a stationary grid affects the:
   A. visibility of grid lines.
   B. efficiency of the grid in cleaning up scatter radiation.
   C. precision required for grid alignment.
   D. focal range.

10. As a general rule, a grid or Bucky should be used when the part thickness is greater than:
    A. 6 cm.
    B. 8 to 10 cm.
    C. 10 to 12 cm.
    D. 14 cm.

11. Which of the following would result in grid cutoff?
    1. Lateral angulation
    2. SID out of the focal range
    3. Position of the x-ray beam off center to one side of the grid
    A. 1 and 2
    B. 1 and 3
    C. 2 and 3
    D. 1, 2, and 3

12. Which of the following will reduce scatter radiation?
    1. Using an air gap
    2. Increasing the kVp
    3. Using a smaller field size
    A. 1 and 2
    B. 1 and 3
    C. 2 and 3
    D. 1, 2, and 3

13. In the diagnostic range of kVp settings (50 to 100 kVp), the majority of scattered radiation will be from which interaction with matter?
    A. Compton effect
    B. Coherent scattering
    C. Photoelectric effect
    D. Characteristic radiation

14. Total absorption of an x-ray photon by the atom of the body part it is termed:
    A. the Compton effect.
    B. coherent scattering.
    C. the photoelectric effect.
    D. characteristic radiation.

15. The majority of photons that are scattered will scatter in which direction?
    A. Toward the head
    B. Toward the feet
    C. To the sides of the patient
    D. Back toward the x-ray tube

16. The standard control limit for the collimator on the x-ray tube is that it must be maintained within a range of:
    A. ±2% of the SID.
    B. ±3% of the SID.
    C. ±4% of the SID.
    D. ±5% of the SID.

Exercise 2

Fill in the blanks with T or F to indicate whether each of the following statements is true or false.

1. _____ Higher kVp results in more scattered radiation fog.

2. _____ The effectiveness of a grid is determined by the grid ratio.

3. _____ High-frequency or stationary grids move during the exposure.

4. _____ A grid with strips that are parallel to each other is called a *crosshatch grid*.

5. _____ An air gap with increased OID increases the intensity of scattered radiation at the image receptor (IR).

6. _____ A grid ratio of 12:1 would be used for mobile radiography.

7. _____ The number of lead strips per inch is called the *grid frequency*.

8. _____ ↑ Tissue thickness = ↑ interactions = ↑ scatter = ↑ fog.

9. _____ The patient is the principal source of scattered radiation in radiography.

10. _____ A grid is placed between the patient and the IR.

11. _____ Compton scatter travels in a forward direction only.

12. _____ Scatter radiation fog reduces the visibility of detail.

13. _____ The standard control limit for the x-ray tube's beam alignment is that the tube must be mounted so that the beam is within 1 degree of perpendicular.

14. _____ The collimator and the beam alignment must be checked using two separate quality control tests.

Exercise 3

Answer the following questions.

1. Which type of radiation interaction produces scattered radiation that is characteristic of the subject irradiated?

   _____

   _____

2. List the two factors that affect the volume of tissue irradiated.

   1. _____

   2. _____

3. When the kVp is increased, will the quantity of secondary radiation fog be increased or decreased? Why?

   _____

   _____

4. What is the principal source of scattered radiation that causes fog in radiography?

   _____

   _____

5. State the grid ratio that is typical of a table Bucky.

   _____

6. What is the usual minimum frequency for a stationary grid in an upright grid cabinet?

   _____

   _____

7. What is the typical radiographic appearance of grid cutoff caused by using an SID that is outside the grid's focal range?

   _____

   _____

8. For what radiographic examination is an air gap commonly used instead of a grid?

   _____

9. How might the image of a vertebra on a "spot film" differ from the image of the same vertebra as part of a 35 × 43 cm radiograph of the spine?

_____

_____

_____

_____

10. How would you determine when to use a grid?

_____

_____

_____

Chapter 12

Formulating X-ray Techniques

Exercise 1

Answer the following questions by selecting the best choice.

1. A technique chart provides the following information:
   1. mA.
   2. kVp.
   3. source-image distance (SID).
   A. 1 and 2
   B. 1 and 3
   C. 2 and 3
   D. 1, 2, and 3

2. Which of the following methods is an effective way to obtain a technique chart?
   1. Have each x-ray operator write down the techniques for 1 week.
   2. Request assistance from the film manufacturer's technical representative.
   3. Hire a consultant who is an expert in technique chart preparation.
   A. 1 and 2
   B. 1 and 3
   C. 2 and 3
   D. 1, 2, and 3

3. Manual technique charts are based on patient part measurements obtained using an x-ray caliper. These measurements are expressed as:
   A. depth, in inches.
   B. circumference, in inches.
   C. thickness, in centimeters.
   D. diameter, in millimeters.

4. The kVp that is sufficient to penetrate the body part adequately without excess exposure to the patient is called:
   A. fixed kVp.
   B. optimum kVp.
   C. variable kVp.
   D. manual kVp.

5. What factors need to be considered when selecting the mA station?
   1. Exposure time
   2. Focal spot size
   3. Thickness of the patient part
   A. 1 and 2
   B. 1 and 3
   C. 2 and 3
   D. 1, 2, and 3

6. When selecting a low mA station (100 mA), you should use:
   A. the large focal spot.
   B. the small focal spot.
   C. either the large or small focal spot.

7. The advantage(s) of using a variable kVp technique chart are:
   1. lower overall image contrast.
   2. improved visibility of detail.
   3. ability to make small incremental changes in exposure technique.
   A. 1 and 2
   B. 1 and 3
   C. 2 and 3
   D. 1, 2, and 3

8. Why should the small focal spot be used as much as possible?
   A. It provides better image sharpness.
   B. It provides better contrast.
   C. It reduces anode heat.
   D. It reduces patient motion.

9. How should exposure factors be adjusted when there is the likelihood of motion?
   A. ↑ mA, ↓ exposure time
   B. ↓ mA, ↑ exposure time
   C. ↓ mA, ↓ exposure time
   D. ↑ mA, ↑ exposure time

10. A satisfactory radiograph is made using 5 mAs with an image receptor relative speed (RS) of 400. How many mAs would be necessary to produce a radiograph of similar density if an RS 100 screen is used?
    A. 1.25 mAs
    B. 10 mAs
    C. 15 mAs
    D. 20 mAs

11. Which mA station can be used for most average-size patients to take advantage of the small focal spot?
    A. 50
    B. 100
    C. 200
    D. 400

12. If 10 mAs produces satisfactory results with a 5:1 ratio grid, what mAs would be needed if a 16:1 ratio grid is used?
    A. 10 mAs
    B. 15 mAs
    C. 20 mAs
    D. 35 mAs

13. Radiography of a wet plaster cast will require an increase in mAs of how much?
    A. 2×
    B. 3×
    C. 4×
    D. 5×

14. A fiberglass cast will require an increase in mAs of how much?
    A. 2×
    B. 3×
    C. Increase 50%
    D. No change required

15. Which of the following x-ray projections can benefit from the use of compensating filters?
    A. Anteroposterior (AP) thoracic spine
    B. Axiolateral hip
    C. AP skull
    D. Both A and B

16. (True/False) Once established on the technique chart, the kVp should never be changed unless contrast needs to be changed.

17. (True/False) If a compensating filter is used with a body part that has significantly varying tissue density, such as the shoulder in AP projection, two separate exposures will still have to be made.

18. (True/False) The use of compensating filters can help reduce the entrance skin exposure.

Exercise 2

Indicate the correct mAs for the new SID to maintain density.

1. If 25 mAs at 40 inches, calculate the mAs at 80 inches.

2. If 30 mAs at 60 inches, calculate the mAs at 30 inches.

3. If 100 mAs at 50 inches, calculate the mAs at 100 inches.

4. If 25 mAs at 30 inches, calculate the mAs at 60 inches.

5. If 100 mAs at 100 inches, calculate the mAs at 50 inches.

Exercise 3

Label the following with an up arrow (↑) to indicate the need for increased technique and a down arrow (↓) to indicate the need for decreased technique.

1. _____ Paget disease

2. _____ Edema

3. _____ Bowel obstruction

4. _____ Sarcoma

5. _____ Hemothorax

6. _____ Pneumothorax

7. _____ Bronchiectasis

8. _____ Advanced age

9. _____ Degenerative arthritis

10. _____ Gout

11. _____ Atelectasis

12. _____ Chronic obstructive pulmonary disease (COPD)

13. _____ Metastases

14. _____ Pleural effusion

Exercise 4

Answer the following questions.

1. Using the technique chart from your facility or the one provided in Appendix B, state the exposure factors for a lateral chest radiograph on a patient measuring 32 cm.

   _____

   _____

2. Which tool and which units are used to measure body part thickness for radiography?

   _____

   _____

3. List steps to take in preparation for making a new exposure technique chart.

   _____

   _____

   _____

   _____

   _____

   _____

4. Using the table of optimum kVp ranges in Appendix C, state the optimum kVp ranges for AP projections of the cervical spine, thoracic spine, and lumbar spine.

_____

_____

_____

5. Assume that your x-ray control panel has the following mA settings: 50, 100, 200, and 300. Which might you use for radiography of the elbow? The lumbar spine? The chest?

_____

_____

_____

_____

6. You are about to take a radiograph that requires 10 mAs and you have decided to use 100 mA. What should the exposure time setting be?

_____

7. List two conditions that require an exposure increase and two that require a decrease.

Increase:

1. _____

2. _____

Decrease:

1. _____

2. _____

8. An acceptable radiograph is made using 200 mA, 0.3 sec, and 70 kVp. Calculate a new exposure that will provide more latitude and less patient dose for the same examination on the same patient.

_____

_____

_____

_____

9. If a satisfactory radiograph is made using 20 mAs at 40 inches SID, what mAs is necessary to produce a similar radiograph at 72 inches SID?

_____

_____

_____

_____

10. A satisfactory radiograph is made using 10 mAs and 76 kVp with a 10:1 grid. How would you change the technique to perform the same examinations without a grid?

_____

_____

_____

_____

Chapter 13

Radiobiology and Radiation Safety

Exercise 1

Answer the following questions by selecting the best choice.

1. The conventional (British system) radiation unit for measuring patient dose is the:
   A. roentgen.
   B. rad.
   C. rem.
   D. sievert.

2. The unit of the conventional system used to measure the radiation exposure in air is:
   A. the roentgen.
   B. C/kg.
   C. the rad.
   D. the gray.

3. The unit commonly used to report occupational dose to radiation workers in the United States is the:
   A. roentgen.
   B. rad.
   C. rem.
   D. gray.

4. According to the Bergonié-Tribondeau law, which of the following types of cells are most radiosensitive?
   A. Skin cells
   B. Nerve and muscle cells
   C. Embryonic tissue
   D. Cells of the gastric mucosa

5. Which of the following types of radiation effects is typical of the risk to a patient undergoing a low-dose, diagnostic x-ray examination?
   A. Short-term effects
   B. Genetic effects
   C. Nonstochastic effects
   D. Stochastic effects

6. Which of the following are nonstochastic radiation effects?
   1. Seizures followed by coma
   2. Erythema
   3. Radiation sickness
   A. 1 and 2
   B. 1 and 3
   C. 2 and 3
   D. 1, 2, and 3

7. The reduction of a limited operator's exposure to ionizing radiation can be accomplished by:
   1. decreasing the time in the radiation field.
   2. increasing the distance from the radiation source.
   3. using low-kVp exposure techniques.
   A. 1 and 2
   B. 1 and 3
   C. 2 and 3
   D. 1, 2, and 3

8. The equivalent dose limit for a whole body dose of occupational radiation exposure for nonpregnant workers over the age of 18 involved in radiation use is:
   A. 5.0 rem per year.
   B. 5.0 mrem per year.
   C. 0.5 mrem per quarter.
   D. 0.5 rem per year.

9. Which of the following are considered low-dose techniques?
   1. Increasing kVp, decreasing mAs
   2. Using slow intensifying screens
   3. Using a minimum source-image distance (SID) of 40 inches
   A. 1 and 2
   B. 1 and 3
   C. 2 and 3
   D. 1, 2, and 3

10. Which of the following changes will decrease patient dose?
    A. Using a slower screen
    B. Decreasing the filtration
    C. Using high-kVp techniques
    D. Using a 36-inch SID

11. When radiation exposure occurs during pregnancy, the greatest risk of birth defects occurs when the dose to the uterus exceeds:
    A. 2 rad.
    B. 5 rad.
    C. 10 rad.
    D. 15 rad.

12. Limited operators can reduce radiation risk to their patients by:
    1. minimizing repeat exposures.
    2. using low-kVp techniques.
    3. collimating closely to the part.
    A. 1 and 2
    B. 1 and 3
    C. 2 and 3
    D. 1, 2, and 3

13. The amount of x-ray energy that is absorbed in the irradiated tissues of the body is termed the:
    A. biologic damage.
    B. quality factor.
    C. absorbed dose.
    D. dose equivalent.

14. If the conventional system states an absorbed dose of 10 rad, the new Système International (SI system) would state this amount as:
    A. 0.10 Gy.
    B. 0.10 Sv.
    C. 100 Gy.
    D. 100 Sv.

15. If the conventional system states an equivalent dose of 26 rem, the new SI system would state this amount as:
    A. 0.26 Gy.
    B. 260 Gy.
    C. 0.26 Sv.
    D. 260 Sv.

16. The greatest cause of unnecessary radiation exposure to patients that can be controlled by the limited operator is:
    A. motion.
    B. repeat exposures.
    C. use of high-kVp techniques.
    D. use of high-mA techniques.

17. Whenever the gonads are within _____ of the margin of the radiation field, gonad dose will be significantly reduced.
    A. 2 cm
    B. 4 cm
    C. 5 cm
    D. 6 cm

18. A pregnant radiation worker's monthly dose equivalent limit is:
    A. 0.01 rem.
    B. 0.05 rem.
    C. 0.10 rem.
    D. 0.50 rem.

19. A 33-year-old radiation worker would have a cumulative dose limit of:
    A. 5 rem.
    B. 10 rem.
    C. 20 rem.
    D. 33 rem.

20. An *erythema* can occur on a patient if the radiation dose to the skin reaches:
    A. 100 rad.
    B. 150 rad.
    C. 200 rem.
    D. 250 rem.

21. (True/False) The standard lead equivalency of the lead aprons used in the radiology department should be a minimum of 0.75 mm lead.

22. (True/False) Radiographers should perform lead apron and glove inspection every 6 months.

23. (True/False) A human who receives an acute whole body exposure of 600 rem (6.0 Sv) will die.

24. (True/False) The earliest biologic effect that will be seen in the human body after exposure to radiation will be nausea and vomiting.

Exercise 2

Match the following terms with their definitions or descriptions.

1. _____ SSD

2. _____ Rad

3. _____ Nonstochastic

4. _____ Roentgen

5. _____ Equivalent dose

6. _____ Carcinogenesis

7. _____ ALARA

8. _____ Mutation

9. _____ Gonad shield

10. _____ Erythema

11. _____ Entrance skin exposure (ESE)

A. Radiation burn
B. Distance from radiation source (x-ray tube) to patient
C. Genetic changes or effects
D. Device to prevent unnecessary radiation to reproductive organs
E. Proportional in severity to the dose of radiation
F. Unit measuring absorbed dose
G. Whole body dose
H. Conventional unit of radiation exposure
I. Radiation exposure should be limited to the lowest possible levels
J. Development of malignant disease
K. Exposure at the skin level

Exercise 3

Answer the following questions.

1. State the SI equivalents for the conventional units R, rad, and rem.

   R _____

   rad _____

   rem _____

2. A radiation worker receives 1 rad of x-ray exposure, 1 rad of thermal neutron exposure, and 1 rad of fast neutron exposure. State the total dose in both rads and rems.

   _____

   _____

3. Using the dose graph in Appendix E, calculate the entrance skin exposure for an exposure of 20 mAs and 80 kVp at 60 inches SSD.

   _____

   _____

4. Explain the difference between long-term and short-term somatic effects of radiation.

_____

_____

_____

_____

_____

_____

5. Describe the risks involved in an x-ray examination of the knee as you would explain it to a patient.

_____

_____

_____

_____

_____

_____

6. At what radiation dose would you see the first signs of a biologic effect? What would that effect be? At what acute dose would death occur?

_____

_____

_____

_____

_____

_____

7. List the common regulatory requirements for gonad shielding. What is its purpose?

_____

_____

_____

_____

_____

_____

8. What should a limited operator do to minimize the need for repeat examinations?

_____

_____

_____

_____

_____

_____

_____

_____

9. What is meant by *low-dose technique?*

_____

_____

_____

_____

10. What is the limited operator's responsibility for ensuring that an embryo is not inadvertently exposed to x-rays?

_____

_____

_____

_____

_____

11. What is the primary method used to provide radiation safety for limited operators?

_____

_____

12. What is the effective dose equivalent limit for nonpregnant workers over age 18? How does this compare with the limit for pregnant women? How is it affected by the ALARA principle?

_____

_____

_____

_____

_____

13. What does ALARA mean?

_____

14. Define *ionizing radiation*.

_____

_____

_____

15. Define *radiation protection*.

_____

_____

_____

16. Where should the radiation badge be worn?

_____

_____

Chapter 14

Introduction to Anatomy, Positioning, and Pathology

Exercise 1

Answer the following questions by selecting the best choice.

1. The study of diseases that cause abnormal changes in the structure or function of body tissues and organs is called:
   A. anatomy.
   B. physiology.
   C. pathology.
   D. inflammation.

2. Which of the following is *not* an example of a tissue?
   A. Neuron
   B. Muscle
   C. Skin
   D. Stomach

3. Bone tissue that has a "honeycomb," or trabecular, structure is called:
   A. cartilage.
   B. marrow.
   C. cancellous tissue.
   D. cortex.

4. The elbow joint is an example of a(n):
   A. synarthrodial joint.
   B. ball and socket joint.
   C. amphiarthrodial joint.
   D. diarthrodial joint.

5. When an extremity is moved toward the central part of the body, this motion is called:
   A. extension.
   B. eversion.
   C. adduction.
   D. abduction.

6. A position in which the patient is lying face up is called:
   A. supine.
   B. anatomic.
   C. prone.
   D. lateral decubitus.

7. When the patient is prone or facing the image receptor (IR), the projection is said to be:
   A. anteroposterior (AP).
   B. posteroanterior (PA).
   C. lateral.
   D. oblique.

8. A disease that is relatively severe and is characterized by a sudden onset and a short duration is said to be:
   A. acute.
   B. chronic.
   C. exogenous.
   D. anomalous.

9. All of the following signs and symptoms may be typical of an inflammatory process except:
   A. pain.
   B. edema.
   C. heat at site.
   D. ischemia.

10. All of the following conditions are classified as a neoplasm except:
    A. carcinoma.
    B. sarcoma.
    C. nosocomial disorder.
    D. lipoma.

Exercise 2

Match the following body systems to the correct descriptors.

1. _____ Integumentary

2. _____ Skeletal

3. _____ Muscular

4. _____ Nervous

5. _____ Endocrine

6. _____ Circulatory

7. _____ Lymphatic

8. _____ Respiratory

9. _____ Digestive

10. _____ Urinary

11. _____ Reproductive

A. Heart and vessels
B. Lungs
C. Skin
D. Lymph nodes, spleen
E. Muscles
F. Kidneys, bladder
G. Hormones
H. Mouth, stomach
 I. Spinal cord
J. Gonads
K. Bones

Exercise 3

Label the fractures in the following figure.

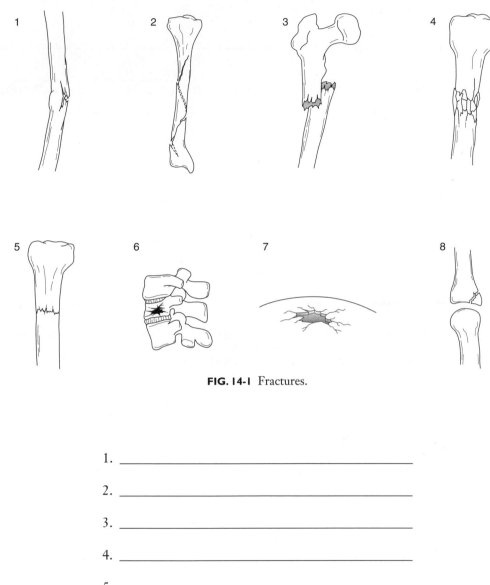

FIG. 14-1 Fractures.

1. _____

2. _____

3. _____

4. _____

5. _____

6. _____

7. _____

8. _____

Exercise 4

Answer the following questions.

1. Name the three main parts of a cell.

    1. _____

    2. _____

    3. _____

2. Name three structures of the body that are composed of connective tissue.

    1. _____

    2. _____

    3. _____

3. What is the difference between a tissue and an organ? _____

    _____

    _____

4. Name two organs that are part of each of the following systems: respiratory, digestive, and urinary.
   Respiratory:

    1. _____

    2. _____

    Digestive:

    1. _____

    2. _____

    Urinary:

    1. _____

    2. _____

5. Describe the function of the skeletal system.

    _____

    _____

6. What is the name of the hard, outer portion of most bones and the inner, honeycomb portion?

    _____

    _____

7. List the three classifications of joints and give an example of each.

   1. _____

   2. _____

   3. _____

8. Define the following terms used to describe joint motion: abduct, adduct, extend, flex, pronate, and supinate.

   _____

   _____

   _____

   _____

   _____

   _____

9. Name the joint that is superior to the knees, inferior to the neck, lateral to the spine, proximal to the hand, and distal to the shoulder.

   _____

10. What is the radiographic term for a body position in which the patient is lying on the left side?

    _____

11. What is the name, and its abbreviation, for the projection in which the central ray enters the anterior surface and exits the posterior surface of the body?

    _____

12. When the patient is lying on the left side and the central ray is vertical, what is the name of the projection?

    _____

13. What phase of respiration does the patient hold for chest radiography? For abdominal radiography?

    _____

14. Since the width of the clavicle is greater than its height, what is the correct IR placement for an AP projection of the clavicle?

    _____

15. List two endogenous conditions and two exogenous conditions.
    Endogenous:

    1. _____

    2. _____

    Exogenous:

    1. _____

    2. _____

16. List the four characteristics of inflammation.

    1. _____

    2. _____

    3. _____

    4. _____

17. Explain the difference between acute and chronic conditions and between benign and malignant conditions.

    _____

    _____

    _____

18. What kinds of conditions are named with terms that end with *-itis* and *-oma*?

    _____

    _____

Chapter 15

Upper Extremity and Shoulder Girdle

Exercise 1
Answer the following questions by selecting the best choice.

1. The small, long bones of the digits are called:
   A. metacarpals.
   B. carpals.
   C. phalanges.
   D. epicondyles.

2. The long narrow bone located anterior to the upper portion of the rib cage and commonly known as the collar bone is the:
   A. humerus.
   B. clavicle.
   C. scapula.
   D. sternum.

3. The bony landmark for wrist positioning that is a prominence on the lateral aspect of wrist is the:
   A. radial head.
   B. scaphoid.
   C. styloid process of the radius.
   D. styloid process of the ulna.

4. The head of the radius articulates with the process on the distal humerus that is called the:
   A. lateral epicondyle.
   B. olecranon process.
   C. trochlea.
   D. capitulum.

5. The use of a stair-step sponge for a posteroanterior (PA) oblique projection of the hand provides better:
   A. patient comfort.
   B. proximity of the digits to the image receptor (IR).
   C. visualization of the interphalangeal joints.
   D. alignment at a precise degree of obliquity.

6. When the limited operator positions the hand for a PA oblique projection using the "modified teacup" position, the anatomic aspect in contact with the IR is:
   A. anteromedial.
   B. anterolateral.
   C. posteromedial.
   D. posterolateral.

7. The PA projection of the wrist in ulnar deviation is an advantageous addition to the routine wrist series in cases of suspected:
   A. Colles fracture.
   B. osteoarthritis.
   C. scaphoid fracture.
   D. posterior dislocation.

8. The projections that constitute a routine examination of the forearm are:
   A. posteroanterior (PA) and lateral.
   B. PA, medial oblique, and lateral.
   C. PA, lateral oblique, and lateral.
   D. anteroposterior (AP) and lateral.

9. When performing a lateral projection of the elbow, it is important to:
   A. flex the elbow 90 degrees.
   B. place the central ray perpendicular to the region of the lateral epicondyle.
   C. place the coronal plane of the humeral epicondyles perpendicular to the IR.
   D. do all of the above.

10. AP projections centered inferior and medial to the coracoid process, with the humerus in both internal and external rotation, constitute a routine examination of the:
    A. scapula.
    B. acromioclavicular joints.
    C. clavicle.
    D. shoulder girdle.

11. When performing a lateral projection of the right scapula, the position of the torso in relation to the IR is:
    A. RPO.
    B. LAO.
    C. RAO.
    D. LPO.

12. Bilateral projections of the shoulders, with and without weights, are used to demonstrate:
    A. acromioclavicular separation.
    B. glenohumeral dislocation.
    C. calcific tendonitis or bursitis.
    D. rotator cuff tears.

13. A PA projection of the shoulder region in which the central ray is directed 30 degrees caudad is taken to demonstrate:
    A. fracture of the proximal humerus.
    B. the clavicle.
    C. the glenohumeral articulation.
    D. the acromioclavicular articulations.

14. To demonstrate a suspected fracture or dislocation in the shoulder region, the radiographic examination should consist of two projections: an AP taken with the coronal plane of the body parallel to the IR, and a(n):
    A. AP projection in external rotation.
    B. AP projection in internal rotation.
    C. transthoracic lateral projection.
    D. Grashey method projection.

15. The fat pad sign may be the only radiographic indication of:
    A. scaphoid fracture.
    B. elbow fracture.
    C. glenohumeral dislocation.
    D. osteomyelitis.

16. The most common type of chronic degenerative joint disease that causes hypertrophy of the bone is:
    A. osteomyelitis.
    B. osteochondroma.
    C. osteoarthritis.
    D. osteoma.

Exercise 2

Label the following illustrations.

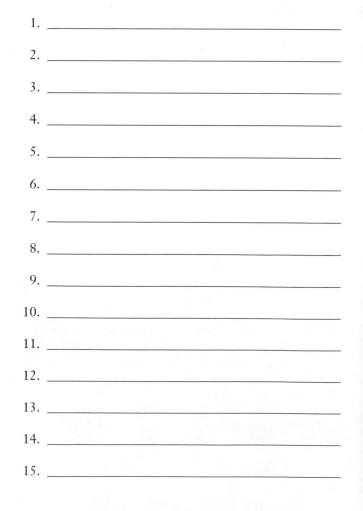

FIG. 15-1 Posterior aspect of hand and wrist.

1. _____

2. _____

3. _____

4. _____

5. _____

6. _____

7. _____

8. _____

9. _____

10. _____

11. _____

12. _____

13. _____

14. _____

15. _____

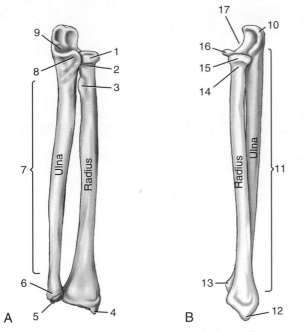

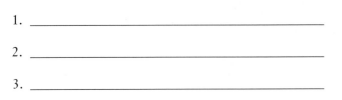

FIG. 15-2 Forearm. **A,** Anterior aspect. **B,** Lateral aspect.

1. _____

2. _____

3. _____

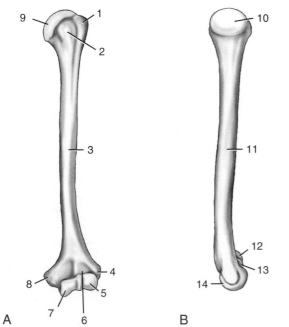

FIG. 15-3 Humerus. **A,** Anterior aspect. **B,** Medial aspect.

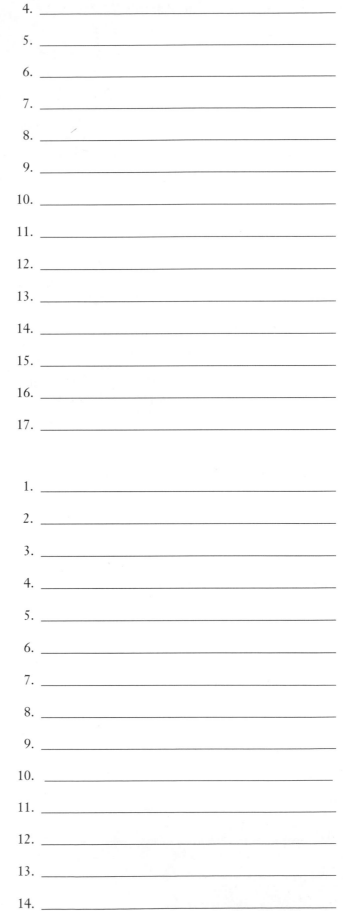

4. _____

5. _____

6. _____

7. _____

8. _____

9. _____

10. _____

11. _____

12. _____

13. _____

14. _____

15. _____

16. _____

17. _____

1. _____

2. _____

3. _____

4. _____

5. _____

6. _____

7. _____

8. _____

9. _____

10. _____

11. _____

12. _____

13. _____

14. _____

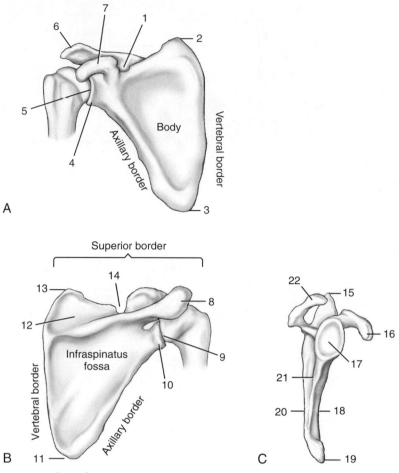

A

B

Superior border

Infraspinatus fossa

Vertebral border

Axillary border

C

FIG. 15-4 Scapula. **A,** Anterior aspect. **B,** Posterior aspect. **C,** Lateral aspect.

1. _____
2. _____
3. _____
4. _____
5. _____
6. _____
7. _____
8. _____
9. _____
10. _____
11. _____

12. _____
13. _____
14. _____
15. _____
16. _____
17. _____
18. _____
19. _____
20. _____
21. _____
22. _____

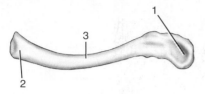

FIG. 15-5 Anterior aspect of clavicle.

1. _____

2. _____

3. _____

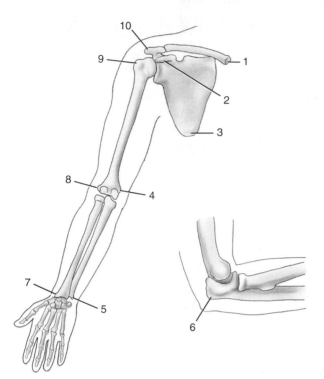

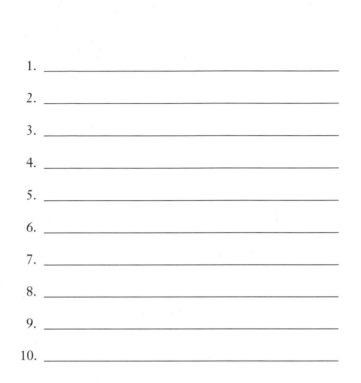

FIG. 15-6 Palpable bony landmarks of upper extremity.

1. _____

2. _____

3. _____

4. _____

5. _____

6. _____

7. _____

8. _____

9. _____

10. _____

Exercise 3

Answer the following questions.

1. Name the middle bone of the third digit and a carpal bone that articulates with the first metacarpal.

_____

2. Is the ulna medial or lateral to the radius?

_____

3. Name the articular processes of the elbow joint.

_____

_____

_____

4. Identify three bony prominences of the scapula.

    1. _____

    2. _____

    3. _____

5. List two ways in which an examination of the thumb differs from an examination of a finger.

    1. _____

    2. _____

6. Describe the differences in positioning for a PA wrist projection and a PA hand projection.

    _____

    _____

    _____

    _____

7. Name two special projections used specifically to demonstrate the scaphoid.

    1. _____

    2. _____

8. Describe the difference between a routine shoulder examination and an examination for an acute injury.

    _____

    _____

    _____

    _____

9. What projections will be performed for an examination of the clavicle?

    _____

    _____

    _____

10. Demonstrate and describe possible arm positions for a lateral projection of the scapula and identify the anatomy visualized on each.

    _____

    _____

    _____

    _____

11. List and describe four commonly seen fractures of the upper extremity.

    1. _____

    2. _____

    3. _____

    4. _____

12. List three general types of nontraumatic pathology that may affect the bones of the upper extremity.

    1. _____

    2. _____

    3. _____

Exercise 4

Label the following images.

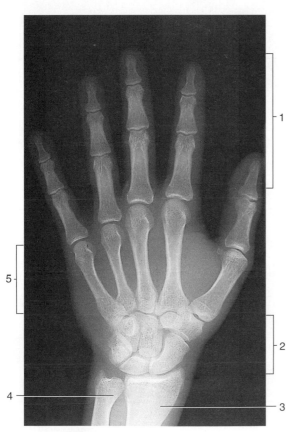

FIG. 15-7 Hand. PA projection.

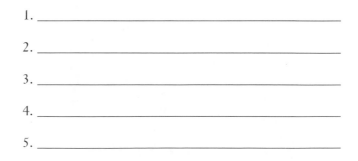

1. _____

2. _____

3. _____

4. _____

5. _____

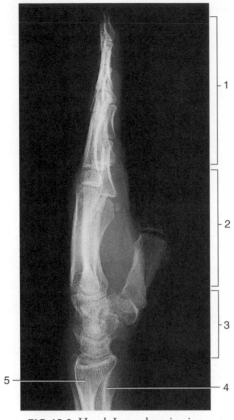

FIG. 15-8 Hand. Lateral projection.

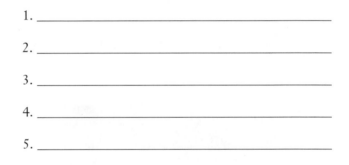

1. _____

2. _____

3. _____

4. _____

5. _____

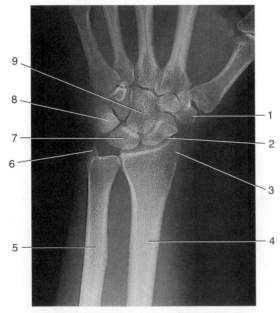

FIG. 15-9 Wrist. PA radiograph.

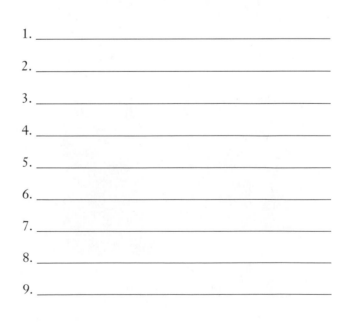

1. _____

2. _____

3. _____

4. _____

5. _____

6. _____

7. _____

8. _____

9. _____

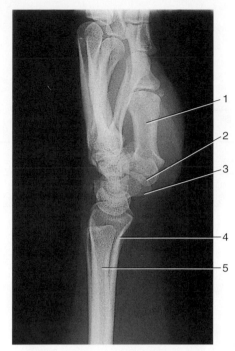

FIG. 15-10 Wrist. Lateral projection.

1. _____

2. _____

3. _____

4. _____

5. _____

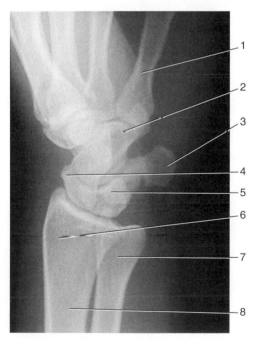

FIG. 15-11 Wrist. AP oblique projection.

1. _____

2. _____

3. _____

4. _____

5. _____

6. _____

7. _____

8. _____

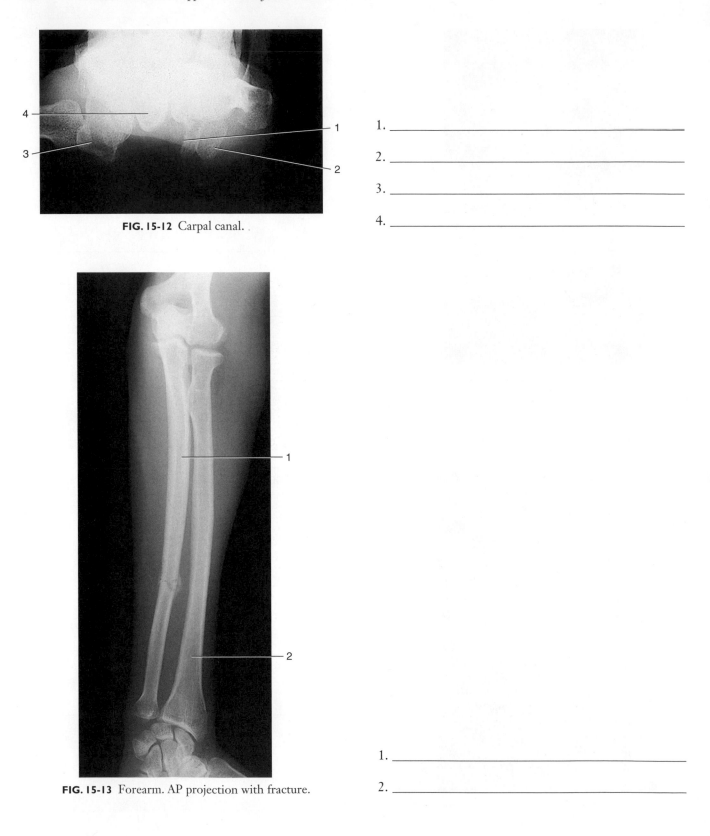

FIG. 15-12 Carpal canal.

1. _____

2. _____

3. _____

4. _____

FIG. 15-13 Forearm. AP projection with fracture.

1. _____

2. _____

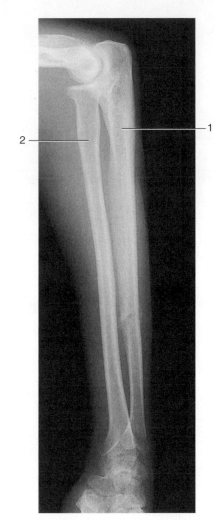

FIG. 15-14 Forearm. Lateral projection with fracture.

1. _____

2. _____

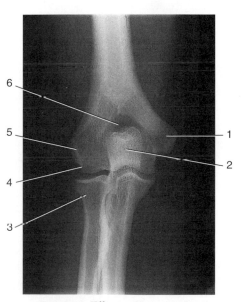

FIG. 15-15 Elbow. AP projection.

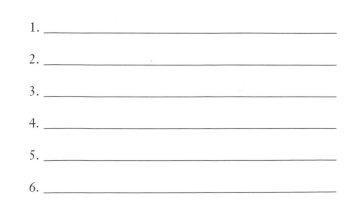

1. _____

2. _____

3. _____

4. _____

5. _____

6. _____

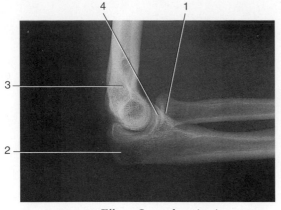

FIG. 15-16 Elbow. Lateral projection.

1. _____

2. _____

3. _____

4. _____

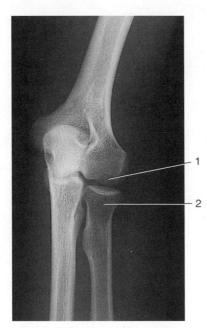

FIG. 15-17 Elbow. AP oblique projection.

1. _____

2. _____

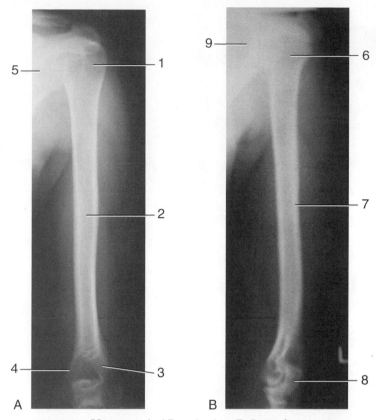

FIG. 15-18 Humerus. **A,** AP projection. **B,** Lateral projection.

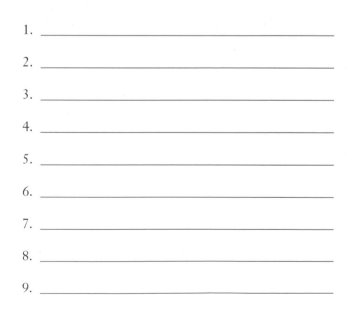

1. _____

2. _____

3. _____

4. _____

5. _____

6. _____

7. _____

8. _____

9. _____

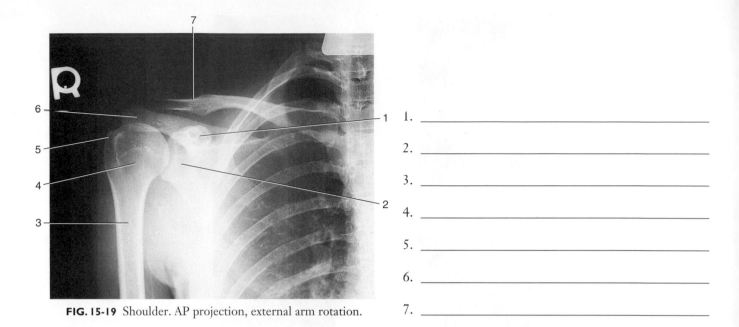

FIG. 15-19 Shoulder. AP projection, external arm rotation.

1. _____

2. _____

3. _____

4. _____

5. _____

6. _____

7. _____

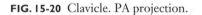

FIG. 15-20 Clavicle. PA projection.

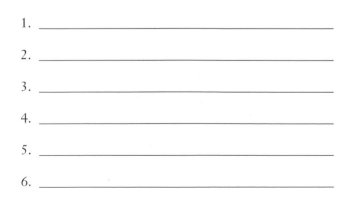

1. _____

2. _____

3. _____

4. _____

5. _____

6. _____

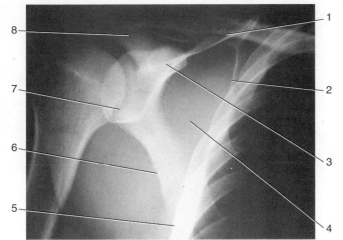

FIG. 15-21 Scapula. AP projection.

1. _____

2. _____

3. _____

4. _____

5. _____

6. _____

7. _____

8. _____

Chapter 16

Lower Extremity and Pelvis

Exercise 1

Answer the following questions by selecting the best choice.

1. The bones of the midfoot consist of the:
   A. phalanges.
   B. tarsals.
   C. metatarsals.
   D. sesamoid bones.

2. Small, flat, oval bones in the region of the first metatarsophalangeal joint are called:
   A. phalanges.
   B. tarsals.
   C. metatarsals.
   D. sesamoid bones.

3. The sesamoid bone that is anterior to the distal femur and is commonly known as the *kneecap* is the:
   A. fibula.
   B. tibia.
   C. patella.
   D. fabella.

4. The ilium, ischium, and pubis join to form a synarthrodial joint at the:
   A. acetabulum.
   B. ilium.
   C. pubic symphysis.
   D. sacroiliac joint.

5. The palpable positioning landmark on the anterior aspect of the lateral pelvis above the hip is called the:
   A. anterior superior iliac spine.
   B. pubic symphysis.
   C. greater trochanter.
   D. ischial tuberosity.

6. When performing an anteroposterior (AP) projection of the foot, the central ray is directed:
   A. 10 degrees toward the toes.
   B. 10 degrees toward the heel.
   C. 15 degrees toward the heel.
   D. perpendicular to the image receptor (IR).

7. When the leg is extended, the ankle is dorsiflexed to form an angle of 90 degrees between foot and leg, the leg is rotated medially approximately 15 to 20 degrees, and the central ray is perpendicular to the IR through the midpoint between the malleoli, the resulting image will demonstrate:
   A. an axial projection of the calcaneus.
   B. a medial oblique projection of the tarsals and metatarsals.
   C. the ankle mortise.
   D. the cuboid and the third cuneiform.

8. When the leg is extended in the supine position, the foot is maximally dorsiflexed, and the central ray is directed 40 degrees cephalad through the sole of the foot, the resulting image will demonstrate:
   A. an axial projection of the calcaneus.
   B. a medial oblique projection of the tarsals and metatarsals.
   C. the cuboid and the third cuneiform.
   D. distal portions of tibia and fibula.

9. A central ray that is angled 5 to 7 degrees cephalad is used when taking:
   A. an AP projection of the ankle.
   B. a lateral projection of the knee.
   C. an AP projection of the foot.
   D. an axial projection of the calcaneus.

10. When the patient is prone, the knee is flexed to form an angle of 75 to 80 degrees between the femur and the lower leg, and the central ray is directed approximately 15 to 20 degrees cephalad through the inferior margin of the patella, the resulting radiograph will demonstrate:
    A. a tangential projection of the patella.
    B. the patella in profile.
    C. the patellofemoral joint.
    D. all of the above.

11. When there is suspicion of a fracture of the patella, flexion of the knee joint for the lateral projection should be limited to:
    A. 5 to 7 degrees.
    B. 10 degrees.
    C. 20 to 30 degrees.
    D. 30 to 45 degrees.

12. When an AP projection of the proximal femur is performed, the IR should be placed so that the:
    A. superior margin is at the level of the greater trochanter.
    B. superior margin is at the level of the iliac crest.
    C. superior margin is at the level of the anterior superior iliac spine.
    D. center is aligned to the midfemur.

13. When an AP projection of the pelvis is performed and there is not a suspicion of a recent fracture, the femurs are:
    A. rotated laterally 15 degrees.
    B. rotated medially 15 degrees.
    C. abducted maximally.
    D. maintained in a neutral AP position.

14. When a lateral projection is needed in cases of a known or suspected hip fracture, which projection(s) would be substituted for the "frog-leg" position?
    A. Axiolateral projection (Danelius-Miller method)
    B. Cross-table lateral projection
    C. Surgical lateral projection
    D. All of the above

15. A systemic disorder that increases the uric acid content of the blood and may cause a joint condition that commonly affects the feet (particularly the joints of the great toe) is called:
    A. osteoarthritis.
    B. gout.
    C. rheumatoid arthritis.
    D. osteoporosis.

16. _____ may cause degeneration of any of the joints of the lower extremity but is most common in the knee and the hip.
    A. Osteoarthritis
    B. Osteomyelitis
    C. Osteogenic sarcoma
    D. Osteoporosis

Exercise 2

Answer the following questions.

1. How many phalanges are there in the great toe? The second toe?

    _____

    _____

2. Is the fibula medial or lateral to the tibia?

    _____

3. Name the bones that form the knee joint.

    _____

    _____

4. Name and point to three bony prominences on your own pelvis.

    1. _____

    2. _____

    3. _____

5. List two ways in which an examination of the foot differs from an examination of the ankle.

1. _____

_____

2. _____

_____

6. Describe the position of the leg for an AP oblique projection (mortise joint) of the ankle.

_____

_____

_____

7. Name two supplemental projections of the knee.

1. _____

2. _____

8. If there is suspicion of fracture of the patella, what projections should be taken? What precautions should be taken?

_____

_____

_____

9. How does a routine hip examination differ from an examination for possible hip fracture? Why?

_____

_____

_____

_____

_____

_____

_____

_____

10. List and describe four specific types of fractures of the lower extremity and hip.

1. _____

_____

2. _____

_____

3. _____

_____

4. _____

_____

11. List three general types of nontraumatic pathology that may affect the bones of the lower extremity or pelvis.

1. _____

2. _____

3. _____

Exercise 3

Label the following illustrations.

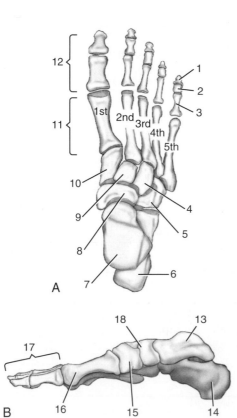

A

B

FIG. 16-1 Foot. **A,** Anterior (dorsal) aspect. **B,** Medial aspect.

1. _____

2. _____

3. _____

4. _____

5. _____

6. _____

7. _____

8. _____

9. _____

10. _____

11. _____

12. _____

13. _____

14. _____

15. _____

16. _____

17. _____

18. _____

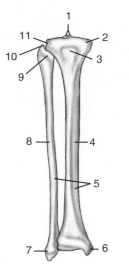
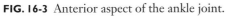
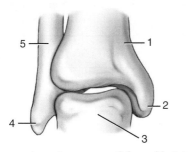

FIG. 16-2 Anterior aspect of the tibia and fibula.

1. _____

2. _____

3. _____

4. _____

5. _____

6. _____

7. _____

8. _____

9. _____

10. _____

11. _____

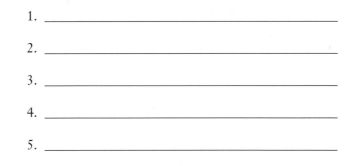

FIG. 16-3 Anterior aspect of the ankle joint.

1. _____

2. _____

3. _____

4. _____

5. _____

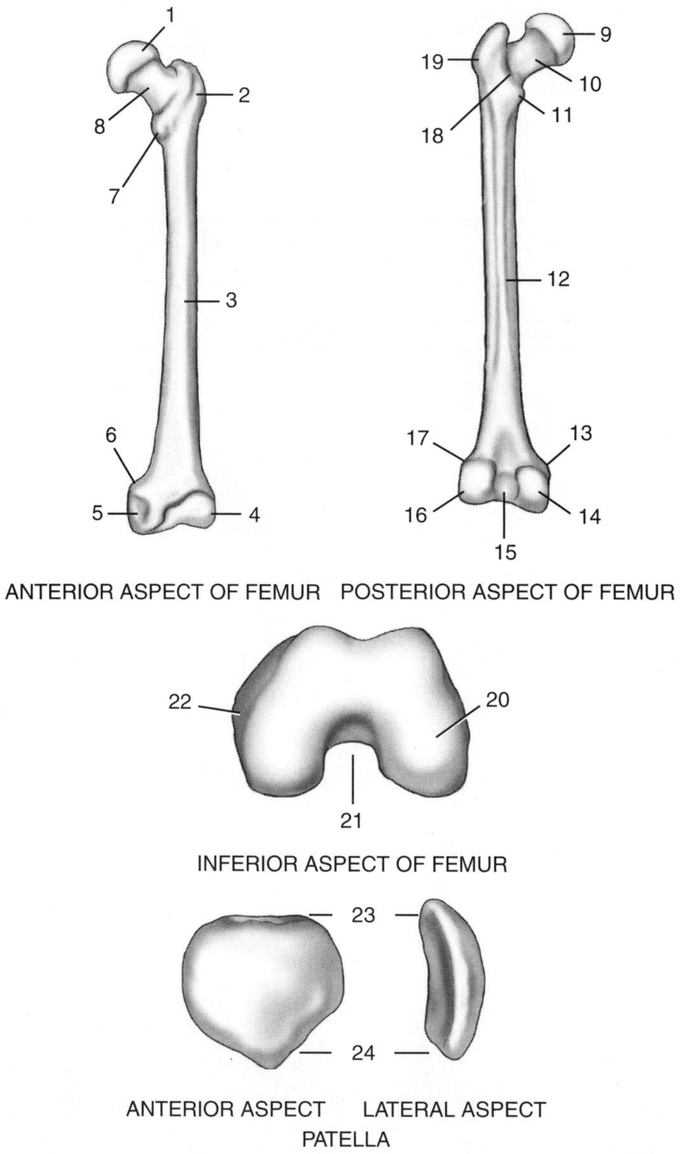

1
2
3
4
5
6
7
8
9
10
11
12
13
14
15
16
17
18
19
ANTERIOR ASPECT OF FEMUR
POSTERIOR ASPECT OF FEMUR
20
21
22
INFERIOR ASPECT OF FEMUR
23
24
ANTERIOR ASPECT
LATERAL ASPECT
PATELLA

FIG. 16-4 Femur and patella.

1. ______________________
2. ______________________
3. ______________________
4. ______________________
5. ______________________
6. ______________________
7. ______________________
8. ______________________
9. ______________________
10. ______________________
11. ______________________
12. ______________________
13. ______________________
14. ______________________
15. ______________________
16. ______________________
17. ______________________
18. ______________________
19. ______________________
20. ______________________
21. ______________________
22. ______________________
23. ______________________
24. ______________________

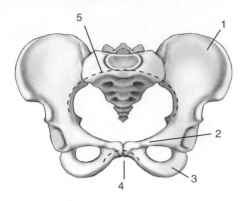

A   FEMALE PELVIS

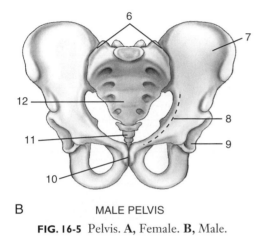

B   MALE PELVIS

FIG. 16-5 Pelvis. **A,** Female. **B,** Male.

1. _____

2. _____

3. _____

4. _____

5. _____

6. _____

7. _____

8. _____

9. _____

10. _____

11. _____

12. _____

Exercise 4

Label the following illustrations.

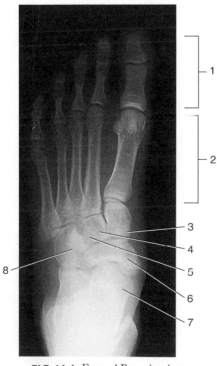

FIG. 16-6 Foot. AP projection.

1. _____

2. _____

3. _____

4. _____

5. _____

6. _____

7. _____

8. _____

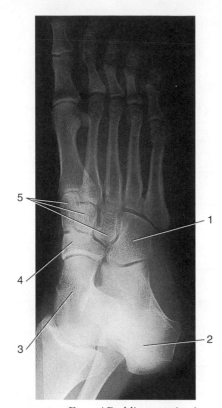

FIG. 16-7 Foot. AP oblique projection.

1. _____

2. _____

3. _____

4. _____

5. _____

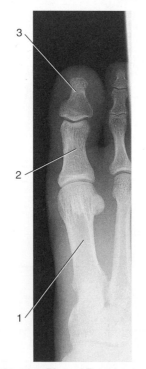

FIG. 16-8 Toes. AP projection.

1. _____

2. _____

3. _____

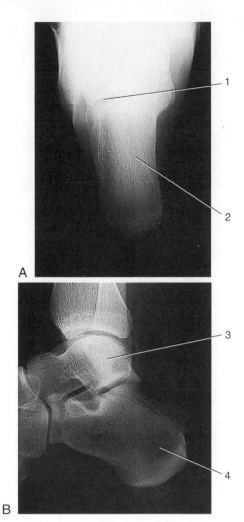

A

B

FIG. 16-9 Calcaneus. **A,** Axial projection. **B,** Lateral projection.

1. _____

2. _____

3. _____

4. _____

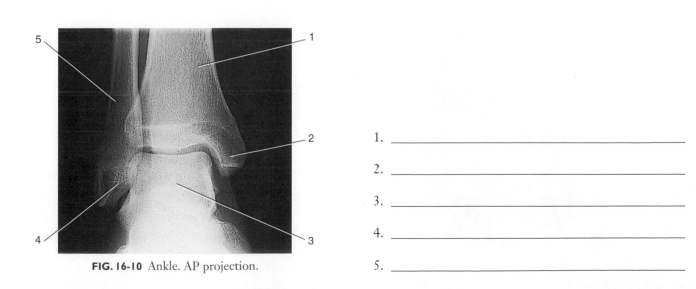

FIG. 16-10 Ankle. AP projection.

1. _____

2. _____

3. _____

4. _____

5. _____

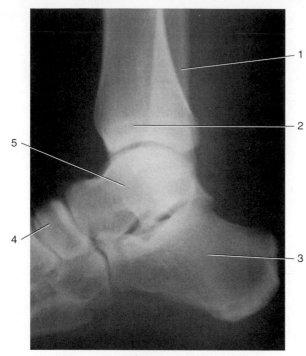

FIG. 16-11 Ankle. Lateral projection.

1. _____

2. _____

3. _____

4. _____

5. _____

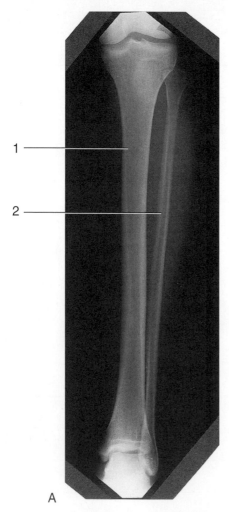

A

FIG. 16-12 Lower leg. **A,** AP projection.

1. _____

2. _____

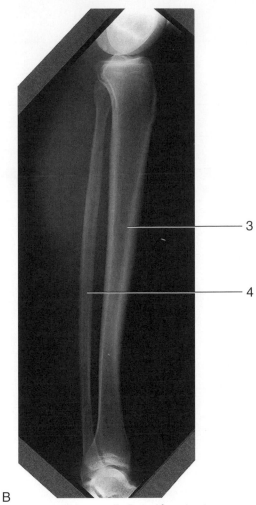

B

FIG. 16-12 Cont'd B, Lateral projection.

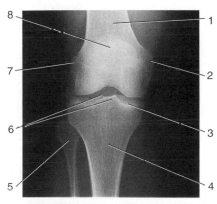

FIG. 16-13 Knee. AP projection.

3. _____

4. _____

1. _____

2. _____

3. _____

4. _____

5. _____

6. _____

7. _____

8. _____

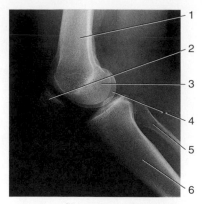

FIG. 16-14 Knee. Lateral projection.

1. _____

2. _____

3. _____

4. _____

5. _____

6. _____

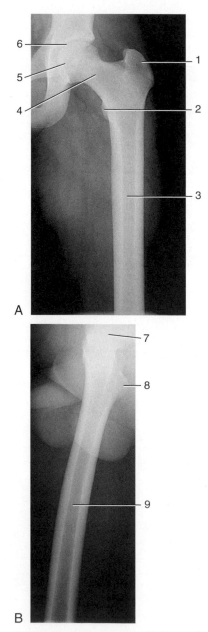

A

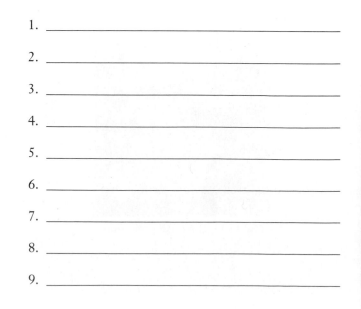

B

FIG. 16-15 Femur. **A,** AP projection. **B,** Lateral projection.

1. _____

2. _____

3. _____

4. _____

5. _____

6. _____

7. _____

8. _____

9. _____

1. _____
2. _____
3. _____
4. _____
5. _____
6. _____
7. _____
8. _____
9. _____
10. _____
11. _____
12. _____
13. _____
14. _____

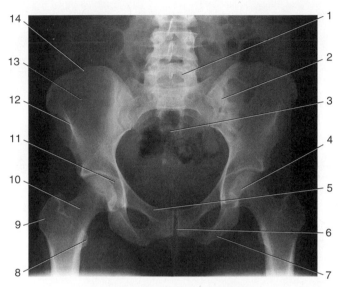

FIG. 16-16 Pelvis symphysis.

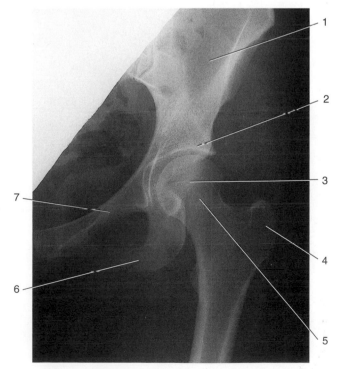

FIG. 16-17 Hip. AP projection.

1. _____
2. _____
3. _____
4. _____
5. _____
6. _____
7. _____

Chapter 17

Spine

Exercise 1

Answer the following questions by selecting the best choice.

1. The region of the spine that consists of five vertebrae and has a lordotic curve is the:
   A. cervical spine.
   B. thoracic spine.
   C. lumbar spine.
   D. sacrum.

2. The articular surfaces of the articular processes of the vertebrae are called:
   A. spinous processes.
   B. transverse processes.
   C. laminae.
   D. facets.

3. The blocklike anterior portion of a typical vertebra is called the:
   A. body.
   B. lamina.
   C. pedicle.
   D. articular process.

4. The number of vertebrae in the normal cervical spine is:
   A. 4.
   B. 5.
   C. 7.
   D. 12.

5. The axis is another name for:
   A. C1.
   B. C2.
   C. T1.
   D. L5.

6. The toothlike projection on which the atlas rotates is called the:
   A. axis.
   B. facet.
   C. articular process.
   D. dens or odontoid process.

7. When an anteroposterior (AP) projection of the cervical spine is performed, the central ray is directed:
   A. perpendicular to the image receptor (IR).
   B. 15 degrees caudad.
   C. 15 degrees cephalad.
   D. 25 degrees cephalad.

8. When the midsagittal plane of the body is parallel to the IR and the central ray is directed perpendicular to C4, the resulting image will be a(n):
   A. AP projection of the lower cervical spine.
   B. lateral projection of the cervical spine.
   C. anterior oblique projection of the cervical spine.
   D. AP projection of the upper cervical spine (open mouth).

9. A shallow breathing technique is used to advantage when taking a lateral projection of the:
   A. cervical spine.
   B. thoracic spine.
   C. lumbar spine.
   D. sacrum.

10. For which of the following projections is it most important to consider the anode heel effect?
    A. AP projection of the lower cervical spine
    B. AP projection of the thoracic spine
    C. Lateral projection the thoracic spine
    D. AP projection of the lumbar spine

11. A supine position with the central ray directed 10 degrees caudad midway between the level of the anterior superior iliac spine and the pubic symphysis is used to demonstrate an:
    A. axial projection of the lumbosacral joint.
    B. AP projection of the view of the sacrum.
    C. AP projection of the coccyx.
    D. AP projection of the pelvis.

12. Spine radiography may be performed with the patient:
    A. upright.
    B. supine.
    C. prone.
    D. all of the above.

13. Patient breathing instructions for all projections of the lumbar spine should include:
    A. suspend breathing on inspiration.
    B. suspend breathing on expiration.
    C. breathe shallowly.
    D. all of the above.

14. The central ray for a lateral projection of the lumbar spine when using a 35 × 43 cm IR is:
    A. perpendicular to the IR through L4.
    B. perpendicular to the IR through L3.
    C. in the midaxillary line.
    D. A and C.

15. The projection commonly called the *swimmer's technique* will demonstrate which region of the spine?
    A. Cervical
    B. Cervicothoracic
    C. Thoracic
    D. Lumbar

16. The positioning steps for the AP projection of the upper cervical spine open-mouth technique include which of the following?
    A. Align the midsagittal plane perpendicular to the IR.
    B. Align the occlusal plane and base of the skull parallel to the horizontal plane.
    C. Use close collimation.
    D. All of the above.

17. Which palpable landmark would be used when positioning for an AP projection of the lumbar spine?
    A. Iliac crest
    B. Jugular notch
    C. Xiphoid process
    D. Lower costal margin

18. When the posterior portions of the neural arch fail to close during early embryonic development, the condition is known as:
    A. spina bifida.
    B. meningomyelocele.
    C. herniated nucleus pulposus.
    D. stenosis.

19. Which region of the spine is the most common site of pathologic compression fracture of vertebral bodies due to osteoporosis?
    A. Cervical
    B. Thoracic
    C. Lumbar
    D. Sacrum

20. Which of the following conditions is demonstrated by magnetic resonance imaging or computed tomography but is not normally seen on routine radiography?
    A. Compression fracture
    B. Spondylosis
    C. Spina bifida
    D. Disk herniation

Exercise 2

Answer the following questions.

1. List the sections of the spine and state the number of vertebrae or vertebral segments in each.

   _____

   _____

   _____

   _____

   _____

2. Which spinal segments have a kyphotic curve? Which have a lordotic curve?

   _____

   _____

   _____

   _____

3. How do the atlas and axis differ from the other cervical vertebrae?

   _____

   _____

   _____

4. On your own body, indicate the location of the mental point, mastoid process, and angle of the mandible, laryngeal prominence, and jugular notch.

   _____

   _____

   _____

   _____

5. An AP projection of the upper cervical spine is unsatisfactory because the patient's upper teeth are superimposed over the atlas and the dens. How should you adjust the position for a satisfactory radiograph?

   _____

   _____

   _____

6. Name and describe positions that will demonstrate each of the following structures: the left cervical intervertebral foramina, the cervical zygapophyseal joints, the lumbar intervertebral foramina, the left lumbar zygapophyseal joints, and the sacroiliac joints.

_____

_____

_____

_____

_____

_____

7. An order for radiographic examination of the cervical spine includes a request for lateral flexion and extension positions. The patient was in a car accident this morning. What precautions are needed? Why?

_____

_____

_____

_____

_____

8. An AP projection of the thoracic spine appears to be quite dark in the region of T1 to T4 and a bit too light in the region of T7 to T12. List possible causes and suggest solutions.

_____

_____

_____

_____

_____

9. How would you instruct a female patient to prepare for a lumbar spine examination?

_____

_____

_____

10. List and describe three common congenital anomalies of the spine.

1. _____

_____

2. _____

_____

3. _____

_____

11. What type of spinal fracture is common among older women with osteoporosis?

_____

12. List two possible causes of nerve root compression and four possible symptoms.
Causes:

1. _____

2. _____

Symptoms:

1. _____

2. _____

3. _____

4. _____

Exercise 3

Label the following illustrations.

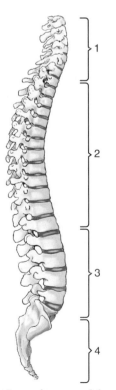

FIG. 17-1 Lateral aspect of the spine.

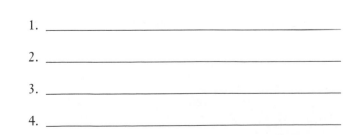

1. _____

2. _____

3. _____

4. _____

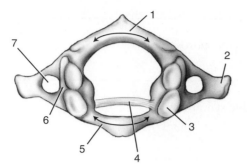

FIG. 17-2 Superior aspect of the atlas (C1).

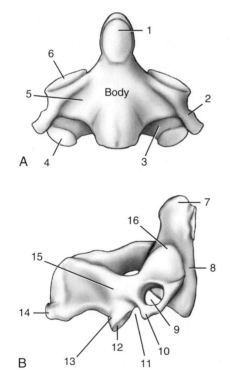

FIG. 17-3 Atlas. **A,** Anterior aspect. **B,** Lateral aspect.

1. _____

2. _____

3. _____

4. _____

5. _____

6. _____

7. _____

1. _____

2. _____

3. _____

4. _____

5. _____

6. _____

7. _____

8. _____

9. _____

10. _____

11. _____

12. _____

13. _____

14. _____

15. _____

16. _____

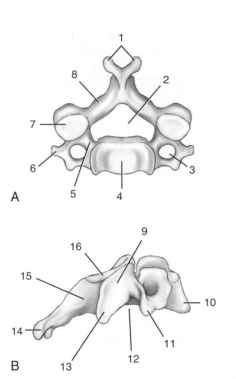

A

B

FIG. 17-4 Typical cervical vertebra. **A,** Superior aspect. **B,** Lateral aspect.

1. _____

2. _____

3. _____

4. _____

5. _____

6. _____

7. _____

8. _____

9. _____

10. _____

11. _____

12. _____

13. _____

14. _____

15. _____

16. _____

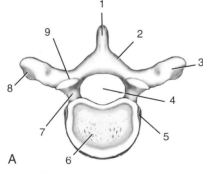

A

FIG. 17-5 Thoracic vertebra. **A,** Superior aspect.

1. _____

2. _____

3. _____

4. _____

5. _____

6. _____

7. _____

8. _____

9. _____

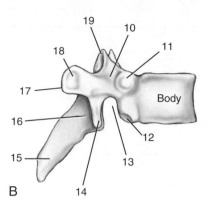

B

FIG. 17-5—cont'd Thoracic vertebra. **B,** Lateral aspect.

10.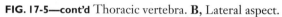

11. _____

12. _____

13. _____

14. _____

15. _____

16. _____

17. _____

18. _____

19. _____

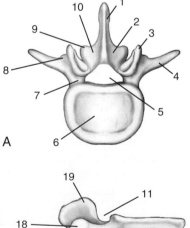

A

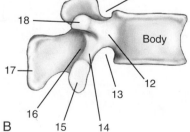

B

FIG. 17-6 Lumbar vertebra. **A,** Superior aspect. **B,** Lateral aspect.

1. _____

2. _____

3. _____

4. _____

5. _____

6. _____

7. _____

8. _____

9. _____

10. _____

11. _____

12. _____

13. _____

14. _____

15. _____

16. _____

17. _____

18. _____

19. _____

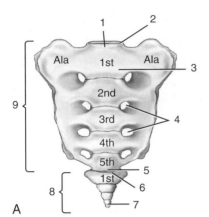

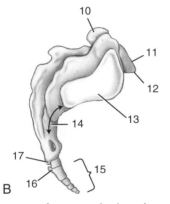

1. _____

2. _____

3. _____

4. _____

5. _____

6. _____

7. _____

8. _____

9. _____

10. _____

11. _____

12. _____

13. _____

14. _____

15. _____

16. _____

17. _____

FIG. 17-7 Sacrum and coccyx. **A,** Anterior aspect. **B,** Lateral aspect.

Exercise 4

Label the following images.

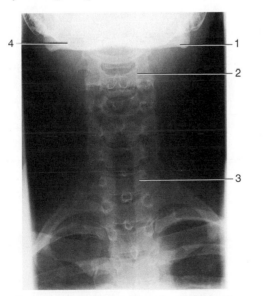

FIG. 17-8 Cervical spine (lower). AP projection.

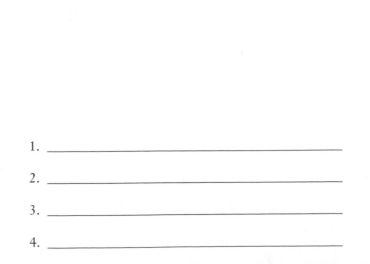

1. _____

2. _____

3. _____

4. _____

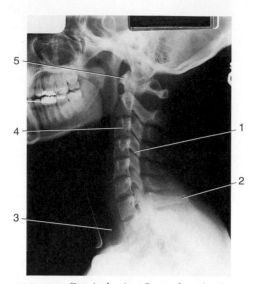

FIG. 17-9 Cervical spine. Lateral projection.

1. _____

2. _____

3. _____

4   _____

5. _____

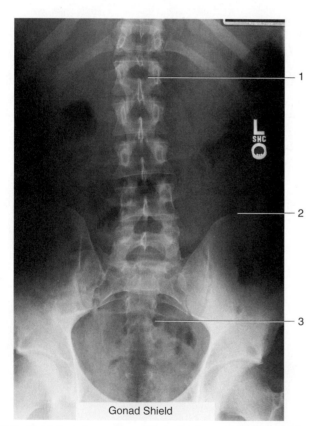

Gonad Shield

FIG. 17-10 Lumbar spine. AP projection, patient recumbent with knees flexed.

1. _____

2. _____

3. _____

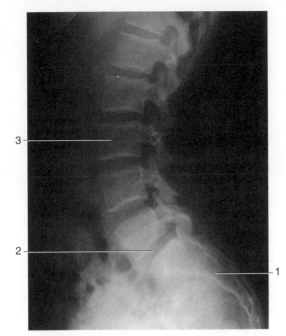

FIG. 17-11 Lumbar spine. Lateral projection.

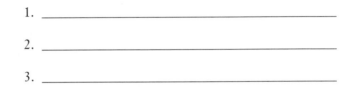

1. _____

2. _____

3. _____

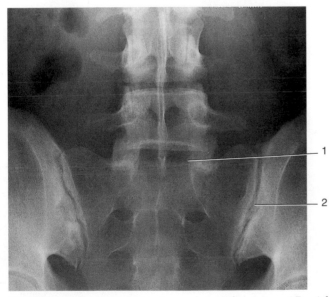

FIG. 17-12 Lumbosacral junction and sacroiliac joints. AP axial projection.

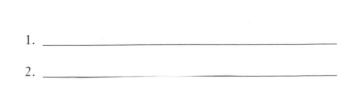

1. _____

2. _____

Chapter 18

Bony Thorax, Chest, and Abdomen

Exercise 1

Answer the following questions by selecting the best choice.

1. Which of the following terms does *not* refer to a portion of the sternum?
   A. Body
   B. Manubrium
   C. Mediastinum
   D. Xiphoid process

2. The lower five pairs of ribs are called:
   A. "true."
   B. "false."
   C. "floating."
   D. cervical.

3. All of the following organs are found within the mediastinum except the:
   A. heart.
   B. lung.
   C. trachea.
   D. ascending aorta.

4. The inferior lateral "corners" of the lungs are called the:
   A. hilum.
   B. inferior lobes.
   C. cardiophrenic angles.
   D. costophrenic angles.

5. When the abdomen is divided into nine regions, the lower middle portion is called the:
   A. hypochondriac region.
   B. iliac region.
   C. hypogastric region.
   D. umbilical region.

6. The first and proximal portion of the small bowel is called the:
   A. duodenum.
   B. pylorus.
   C. jejunum.
   D. ileum.

7. The function(s) of the large intestine include:
   A. reclamation of water from intestinal contents.
   B. eliminate of solid waste.
   C. production of bile.
   D. A and B.

8. Routine projections for the right fourth posterior rib are:
   A. posteroanterior (PA) and left anterior oblique (LAO).
   B. PA and right anterior oblique (RAO).
   C. anteroposterior (AP) and right posterior oblique (RPO).
   D. AP and left posterior oblique (LPO).

9. Routine projections for the left tenth anterior rib are:
   A. PA and LAO.
   B. PA and RAO.
   C. AP and RPO.
   D. AP and LPO.

10. Routine projections for the sternum are:
    A. PA and lateral.
    B. PA and RAO.
    C. Lateral and RAO.
    D. Lateral and LAO.

11. Examination of the chest differs from examination of the ribs in that:
    A. a 72-inch source-image distance (SID) is used.
    B. a higher kVp is used.
    C. exposure is made on expiration.
    D. both A and B.

12. An upright AP projection of the abdomen is useful for the visualization of:
    A. air-fluid levels in the intestines.
    B. liver size.
    C. kidney stones.
    D. diverticulosis.

13. When a PA projection of the chest is performed, the correct SID is:
    A. 40 inches.
    B. 48 inches.
    C. 60 inches.
    D. 72 inches.

14. Lateral projections of the chest are taken with the left side against the image receptor (IR) because:
    A. magnification of the cardiac silhouette is minimized with the left side nearer the IR.
    B. it is conventional to have a routine standard, and the left has been established as the standard.
    C. lung pathology is more common on the left side.
    D. the right hilum provides high-contrast details that may be confusing.

15. Which of the following techniques is desirable for chest radiography?
    A. High kVp, high mA, and short exposure time
    B. Low kVp and 72 inches SID
    C. Low kVp, high mAs
    D. High kVp, 72 inches SID, and low mA

16. Which of the following projections benefits from the use of a "breathing technique"?
    A. PA chest
    B. Oblique ribs
    C. Oblique sternum
    D. Lateral sternum

17. To demonstrate air-fluid levels in radiography, use:
    A. the decubitus position.
    B. the upright position.
    C. a horizontal x-ray beam.
    D. all of the above.

18. Breathing instructions for a PA projection of the chest should include:
    A. suspend breathing on first deep inspiration.
    B. suspend breathing on second deep inspiration.
    C. suspend breathing on first deep expiration.
    D. suspend breathing on second deep expiration.

19. Which of the following conditions is an inflammatory occupational lung disease caused by inhaling irritating dust?
    A. Tuberculosis
    B. Pneumoconiosis
    C. *Pneumocystis carinii* pneumonia
    D. Pneumothorax

20. All of the following abdominal features should be seen on "plain films" (noncontrast media studies) of the abdomen except:
    A. the outer contours the kidneys.
    B. gas in the colon.
    C. the psoas muscle.
    D. the pancreas.

Exercise 2

Answer the following questions.

1. Name the parts of the sternum and point to each on your own body.

    _____

    _____

    _____

    _____

2. Make a simple drawing of a lung and indicate the apex, the hilum, the costophrenic angle, and the cardiophrenic angle.

3. Name four structures located within the mediastinum and state the body system to which each belongs.

   1. _____

   2. _____

   3. _____

   4. _____

4. Name two organs found in each quadrant of the abdomen.

   Right upper quadrant: _____

   Left upper quadrant: _____

   Right lower quadrant: _____

   Left lower quadrant: _____

5. Name the projections that constitute a routine examination of the left upper anterior ribs and the right lower posterior ribs.

   _____

   _____

   _____

6. Should ribs below the diaphragm be exposed on inspiration or expiration?

   _____

7. List as many differences as you can between rib radiography and chest radiography.

   _____

   _____

   _____

   _____

   _____

   _____

   _____

8. If a patient with acute abdominal pain cannot stand for an upright AP abdominal projection, what projection should be substituted? Why is this important?

   _____

   _____

   _____

   _____

9. List three conditions that involve inflammation of the lungs.

   1. _____

   2. _____

   3. _____

10. Name two common radiographic findings in cases of congestive heart failure.

    1. _____

    2. _____

11. What radiographic findings are typical of intestinal obstruction?

    _____

    _____

    _____

12. State two reasons why a chest radiograph might be important for a patient who has severe abdominal pain.

    1. _____

    2. _____

    _____

Exercise 3

Label the following illustrations.

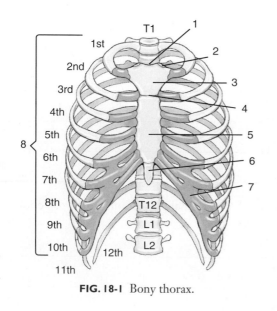

FIG. 18-1 Bony thorax.

1. _____

2. _____

3. _____

4. _____

5. _____

6. _____

7. _____

8. _____

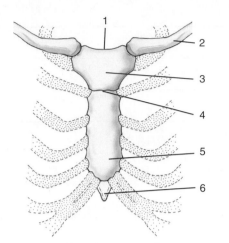

FIG. 18-2 Anterior aspect of sternum.

1. _____

2. _____

3. _____

4. _____

5. _____

6. _____

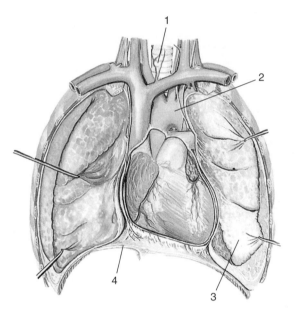

FIG. 18-3 Thoracic cavity.

1. _____

2. _____

3. _____

4. _____

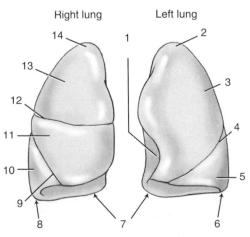

Right lung   Left lung

FIG. 18-4 Anterior aspect of lungs.

1. _____

2. _____

3. _____

4. _____

5. _____

6. _____

7. _____

8. _____

9. _____

10. _____

11. _____

12. _____

13. _____

14. _____

1. _____

2. _____

3. _____

4. _____

5. _____

6. _____

7. _____

8. _____

9. _____

10. _____

11. _____

12. _____

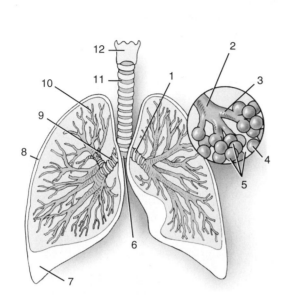

FIG. 18-5 Organs of the respiratory system within the thoracic cavity.

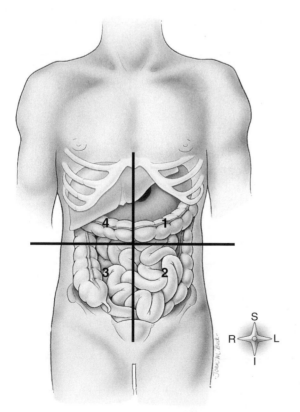

FIG. 18-6 Abdominopelvic cavity divided into quadrants.

1. _____

2. _____

3. _____

4. _____

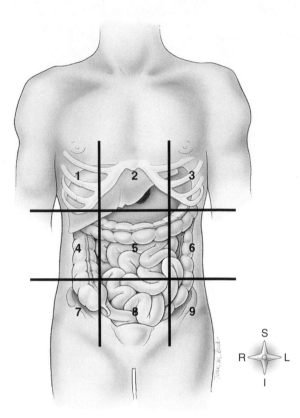

FIG. 18-7 Nine abdominal regions.

1. _____
2. _____
3. _____
4. _____
5. _____
6. _____
7. _____
8. _____
9. _____

1. _____
2. _____
3. _____
4. _____
5. _____
6. _____
7. _____
8. _____
9. _____
10. _____
11. _____
12. _____
13. _____
14. _____
15. _____
16. _____
17. _____
18. _____

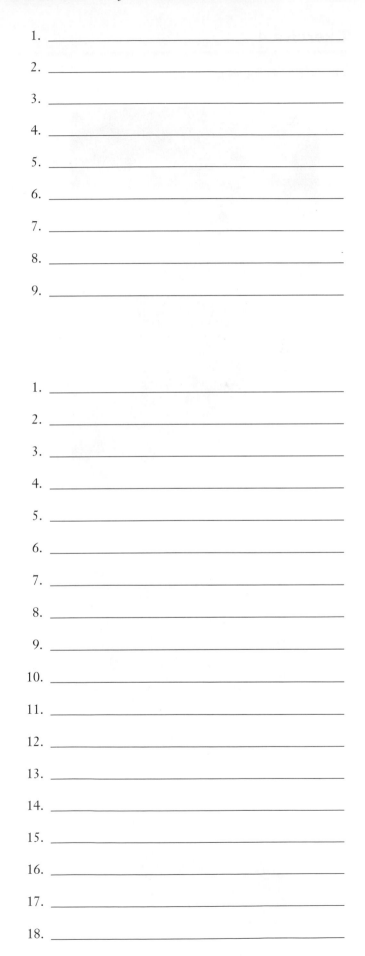

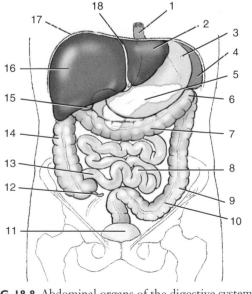

FIG. 18-8 Abdominal organs of the digestive system.

Exercise 4

Label the following images.

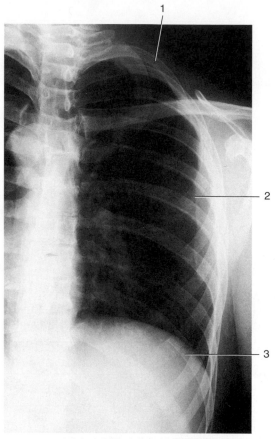

FIG. 18-9 Upper posterior ribs. AP projection.

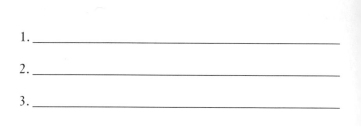

1. _____

2. _____

3. _____

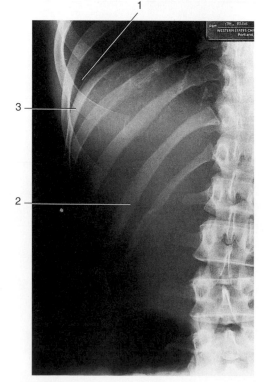

FIG. 18-10 Lower posterior ribs. AP projection.

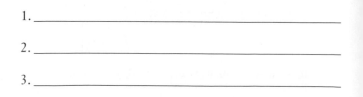

1. _____

2. _____

3. _____

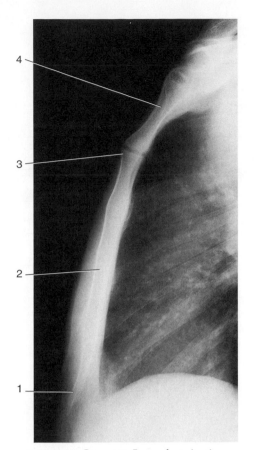

FIG. 18-11 Sternum. Lateral projection.

1. _____

2. _____

3. _____

4. _____

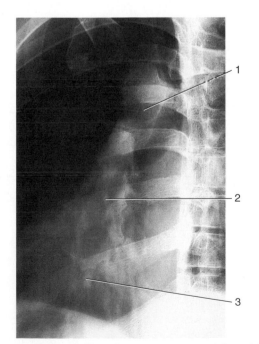

FIG. 18-12 Sternum. PA oblique projection (RAO position).

1. _____

2. _____

3. _____

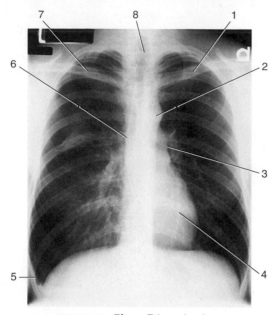

FIG. 18-13 Chest. PA projection.

1. _____

2. _____

3. _____

4. _____

5. _____

6. _____

7. _____

8. _____

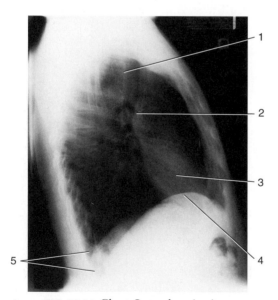

FIG. 18-14 Chest. Lateral projection.

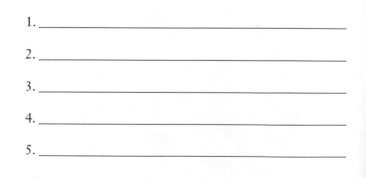

1. _____

2. _____

3. _____

4. _____

5. _____

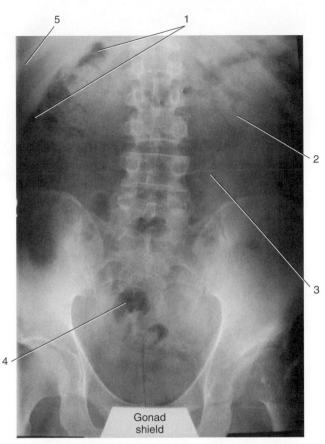

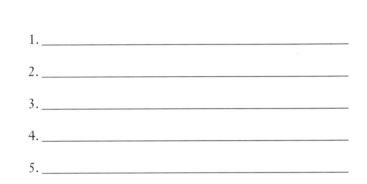

FIG. 18-15 Abdomen. AP projection, patient recumbent.

1. _____

2. _____

3. _____

4. _____

5. _____

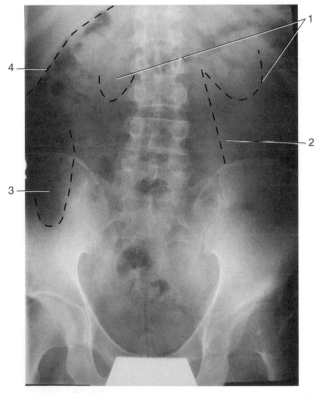

FIG. 18-16 AP abdomen radiograph showing kidney shadows, liver margin, and psoas muscles.

1. _____

2. _____

3. _____

4. _____

Chapter 19

Skull, Facial Bones, and Paranasal Sinuses

Exercise 1

Answer the following questions by selecting the best choice.

1. Which of the following bones is not a part of the cranium?
   A. Parietal
   B. Frontal
   C. Maxillary
   D. Temporal

2. The bony prominence on the frontal bone between the eyebrows is called the:
   A. acanthion.
   B. glabella.
   C. gonion.
   D. nasion.

3. All of the following bones contain paranasal sinuses except the:
   A. frontal bone.
   B. ethmoid bone.
   C. temporal bone.
   D. maxilla.

4. When a posteroanterior (PA) projection of the skull is performed, the central ray is directed:
   A. perpendicular to the film.
   B. 15 degrees cephalad.
   C. 15 degrees caudad.
   D. 30 degrees cephalad.

5. A projection of the skull in which the sagittal plane is parallel to the image receptor (IR) and the interpupillary line is perpendicular to the IR is a(n):
   A. PA projection.
   B. anteroposterior (AP) axial projection (Towne method).
   C. Waters projection.
   D. lateral projection.

6. A lateral projection of the face using detail screens tabletop (nongrid) is used to demonstrate the:
   A. mandible.
   B. zygoma.
   C. orbits.
   D. nasal bones.

7. When the patient is supine, the sagittal plane of the skull is perpendicular to the IR, the orbitomeatal line is perpendicular to the IR, and the central ray is angled 30 degrees caudad, the resulting radiograph will demonstrate the:
   A. frontal bone.
   B. temporal bones.
   C. posterior parietal bones and the occipital bone.
   D. maxillary sinuses.

8. When the right and left halves of the skull do not appear symmetric on a PA or AP projection, this is a sign that:
   A. the neck extended too much.
   B. the neck flexed too much.
   C. the sagittal plane is not perpendicular to the film.
   D. the central ray is not centered to the film.

9. A blow-out fracture involves the:
   A. floor of the orbit.
   B. occipital bone.
   C. mandible.
   D. nasal bones.

10. The projection that will demonstrate all of the paranasal sinuses is the:
    A. lateral projection.
    B. parietoacanthial projection.
    C. PA axial projection.
    D. all of the above.

Exercise 2

Answer the following questions.

1. Name the bones that make up the cranium.

   _____

   _____

   _____

2. Which cranial bones contain the auditory canals?

   _____

   _____

3. List the bones that make up the orbit.

   _____

   _____

   _____

4. List the bones that contain paranasal sinuses.

   _____

   _____

   _____

5. Name a projection that demonstrates the cranial base.

   _____

   _____

   _____

6. Compare the procedure for an AP axial (Towne method) projection with the procedure for demonstrating the
   same structures with the patient prone.

   _____

   _____

   _____

   _____

   _____

7. Name two projections that demonstrate the maxillary sinuses.

   1. _____

   2. _____

8. How does the procedure for a lateral projection of the nasal bones differ from that for a lateral projection of the facial bones?

   _____

   _____

   _____

   _____

   _____

9. Describe the patient/part position for a parietoacanthial (Waters method) projection of the facial bones and sinuses.

   _____

   _____

   _____

   _____

10. If the petrous ridge is projected over the floor of the maxillary sinuses on the parietoacanthial (Waters method) projection, how should the position be modified to clearly demonstrate this area?

   _____

   _____

   _____

   _____

11. List three types of facial fractures and state the projection(s) most likely to provide a clear demonstration of each.

   1. _____

   2. _____

   3. _____

12. Name three types of pathology that may be diagnosed by radiography of the cranium.

   1. _____

   2. _____

   3. _____

Exercise 3

Label the following illustrations.

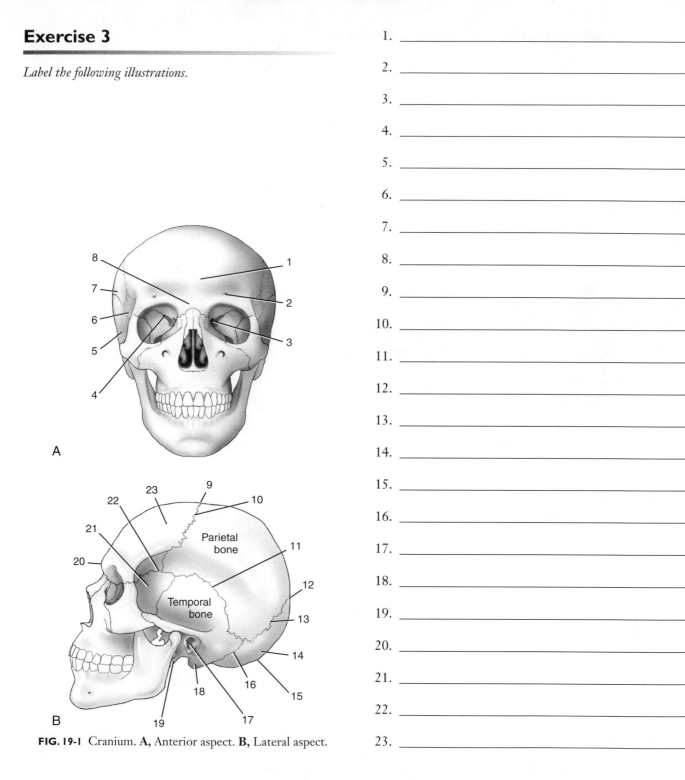

A

B

FIG. 19-1 Cranium. **A,** Anterior aspect. **B,** Lateral aspect.

1. _____
2. _____
3. _____
4. _____
5. _____
6. _____
7. _____
8. _____
9. _____
10. _____
11. _____
12. _____
13. _____
14. _____
15. _____
16. _____
17. _____
18. _____
19. _____
20. _____
21. _____
22. _____
23. _____

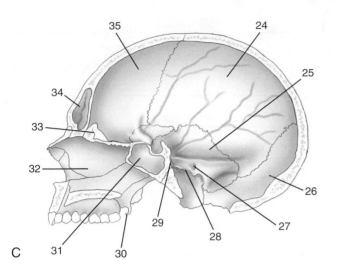

C

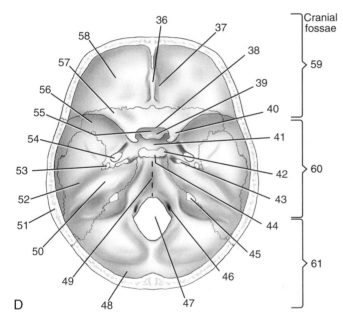

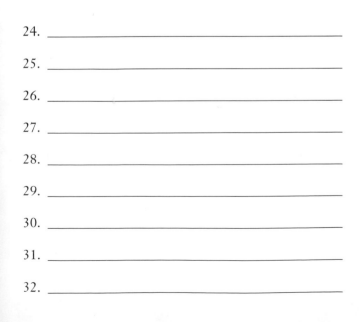

D

FIG. 19-1—cont'd C, Lateral aspect of interior of cranium. **D,** Superior aspect of cranial base.

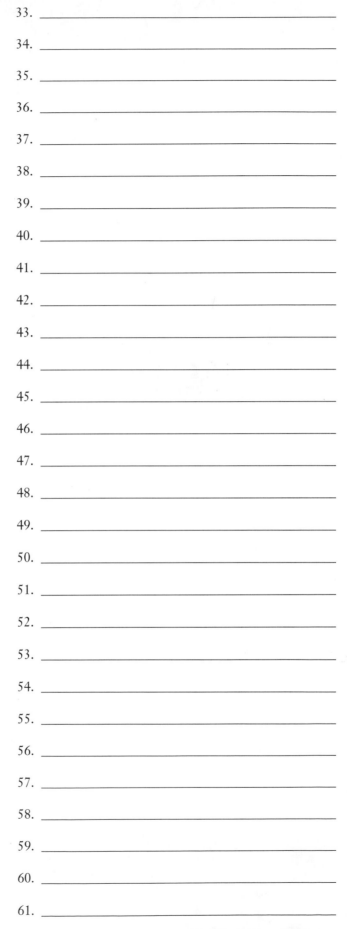

24. _____
25. _____
26. _____
27. _____
28. _____
29. _____
30. _____
31. _____
32. _____

33. _____
34. _____
35. _____
36. _____
37. _____
38. _____
39. _____
40. _____
41. _____
42. _____
43. _____
44. _____
45. _____
46. _____
47. _____
48. _____
49. _____
50. _____
51. _____
52. _____
53. _____
54. _____
55. _____
56. _____
57. _____
58. _____
59. _____
60. _____
61. _____

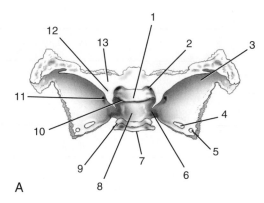

A

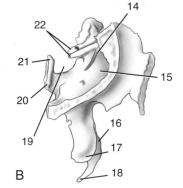

B

FIG. 19-2 Sphenoid bone. **A,** Superior aspect. **B,** Lateral aspect.

1. _____

2. _____

3. _____

4. _____

5. _____

6. _____

7. _____

8. _____

9. _____

10. _____

11. _____

12. _____

13. _____

14. _____

15. _____

16. _____

17. _____

18. _____

19. _____

20. _____

21. _____

22. _____

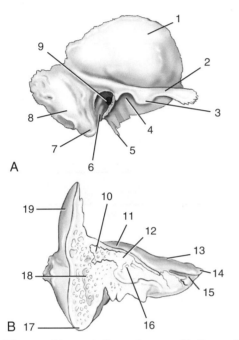

A

B

FIG. 19-3 Temporal bone. **A,** Lateral aspect. **B,** Coronal section through mastoid and petrous portions.

1. _____

2. _____

3. _____

4. _____

5. _____

6. _____

7. _____

8. _____

9. _____

10. _____

11. _____

12. _____

13. _____

14. _____

15. _____

16. _____

17. _____

18. _____

19. _____

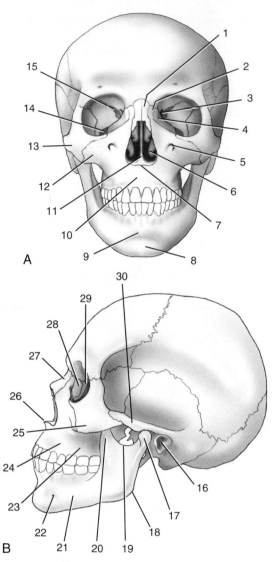

A

B

FIG. 19-4 Facial bones. **A,** Anterior aspect. **B,** Lateral aspect.

6. _____

7. _____

8. _____

9. _____

10. _____

11. _____

12. _____

13. _____

14. _____

15. _____

16. _____

17. _____

18. _____

19. _____

20. _____

21. _____

22. _____

23. _____

24. _____

25. _____

26. _____

27. _____

28. _____

29. _____

30. _____

1. _____

2. _____

3. _____

4. _____

5. _____

31. _____

32. _____

33. _____

34. _____

35. _____

36. _____

37. _____

38. _____

39. _____

40. _____

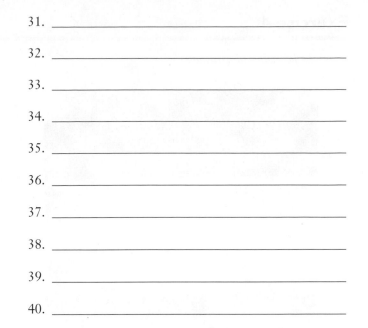

C

FIG. 19-4—cont'd C, Interior of facial bones, lateral aspect.

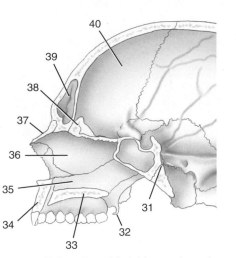

A

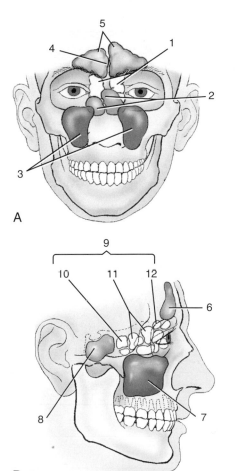

B

FIG. 19-5 Paranasal sinuses. **A,** Anterior aspect. **B,** Lateral aspect.

1. _____

2. _____

3. _____

4. _____

5. _____

6. _____

7. _____

8. _____

9. _____

10. _____

11. _____

12. _____

Exercise 4

Label the following illustrations.

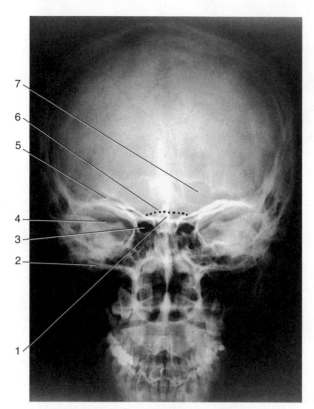

FIG. 19-6 Cranium. PA projection.

1. _____

2. _____

3. _____

4. _____

5. _____

6. _____

7. _____

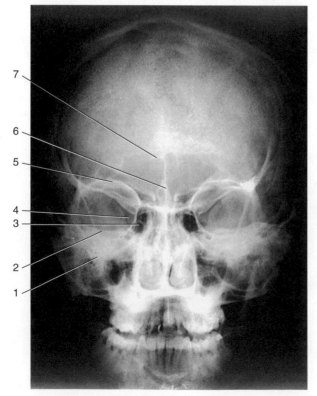

FIG. 19-7 Cranium. PA axial projection.

1. _____

2. _____

3. _____

4. _____

5. _____

6. _____

7. _____

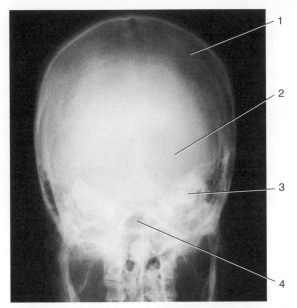
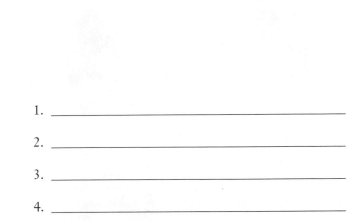

1. _____

2. _____

3. _____

4. _____

FIG. 19-8 Cranium. AP axial projection (Towne method).

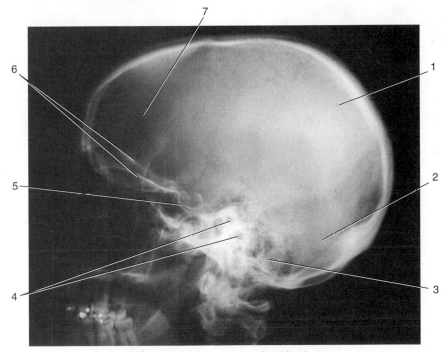
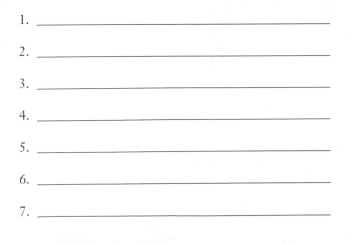

FIG. 19-9 Cranium. Lateral projection.

1. _____

2. _____

3. _____

4. _____

5. _____

6. _____

7. _____

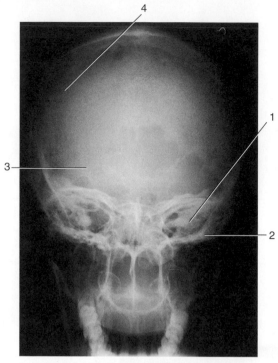
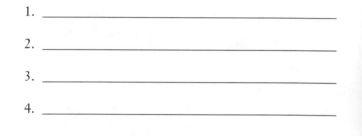
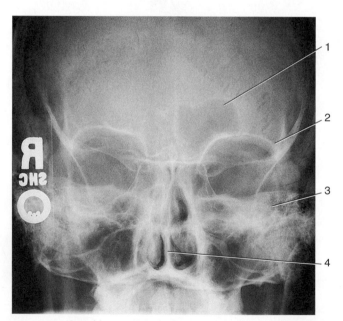
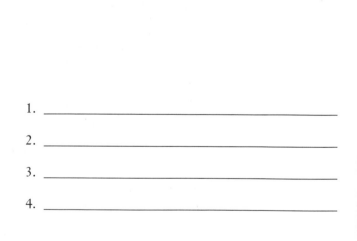

FIG. 19-10 Cranium. AP projection.

1. _____

2. _____

3. _____

4. _____

FIG. 19-11 Facial bones. PA axial projection (Caldwell method).

1. _____

2. _____

3. _____

4. _____

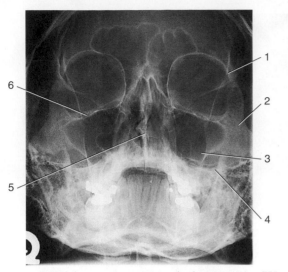

FIG. 19-12 Facial bones. Parietoacanthial projection (Waters method).

1. _____

2. _____

3. _____

4. _____

5. _____

6. _____

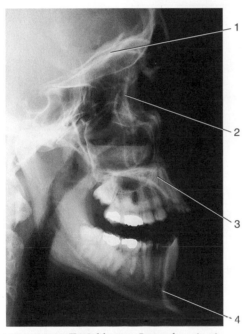

FIG. 19-13 Facial bones. Lateral projection.

1. _____

2. _____

3. _____

4. _____

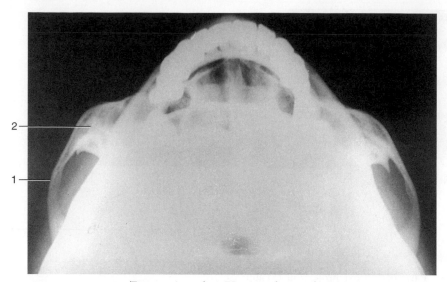

FIG. 19-14 Zygomatic arches. Verticosubmental projection.

1. _____

2. _____

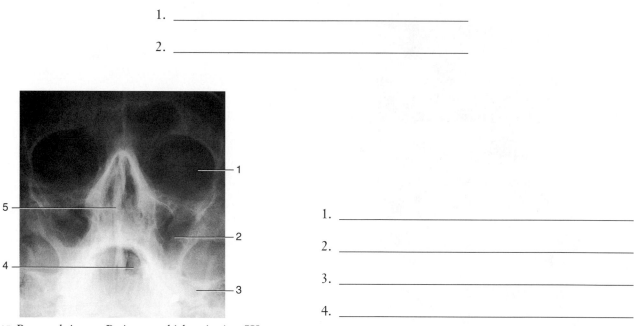

FIG. 19-15 Paranasal sinuses. Parietoacanthial projection (Waters method).

1. _____

2. _____

3. _____

4. _____

5. _____

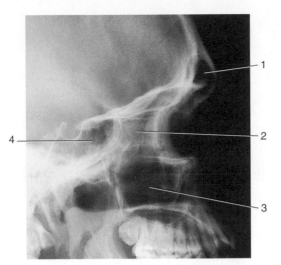

FIG. 19-16 Paranasal sinuses. Lateral projection.

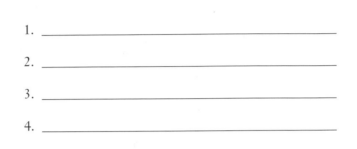

1. _____

2. _____

3. _____

4. _____

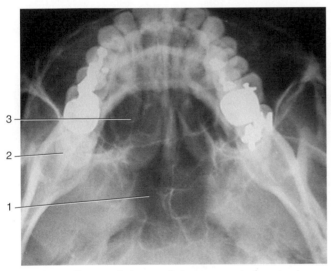

FIG. 19-17 Paranasal sinuses. Submentovertical projection.

1. _____

2. _____

3. _____

Chapter 20

Radiography of Pediatric and Geriatric Patients

Answer the following questions.

1. The term that refers to the care of older adults is _____.

2. The term that refers to the care of infants and children is _____.

3. List three things you might do to calm an infant.

   1. _____

   2. _____

   3. _____

4. (True/False) More information is communicated nonverbally than with words.

5. When a toddler is refusing to cooperate, what are two things you can do that might change the child's attitude?

   1. _____

   2. _____

6. Explain what is meant by a "valid choice."

   _____

   _____

7. (True/False) When a child is to have a radiographic examination, a parent should never be allowed in the x-ray room.

8. (True/False) Mechanical immobilization is preferable to having someone hold a child during an x-ray exposure.

9. (True/False) When a child must be held during an x-ray exposure, x-ray personnel should hold the child.

10. The principal objective when immobilizing an infant or child for radiography is _____
    _____.

11. Bilateral studies of the _____ and the _____ are seldom required for adults, but are usually performed for children.

12. List three ways in which the anatomy of children differs from that of adults.

    1. _____

    2. _____

    3. _____

13. (True/False) Chest radiography on small children does not require the use of a grid.

14. An adult knee measuring 13 cm requires an exposure of 5 mAs and 70 kVp at 40 inches source-image distance, with no grid. Suggest a set of exposure factors that will produce a satisfactory radiograph on a 9-year-old patient whose knee measures 8 cm.

    _____

15. (Circle the correct word.) When making radiographs of small children it is usually advantageous to use a (high/low) mA setting.

16. Why might a physician order frontal chest radiographs on a child to be taken on both inspiration and expiration?

    _____

17. An incomplete fracture in which the periosteum ruptures and the cortex separates on one side of the bone, but the

    other side remains intact, is called a _____ fracture.

18. A common anatomic area for radiography to determine bone age is the

    _____ .

19. Nonaccidental trauma is another term for

    _____ .

20. List five signs in a child that should raise suspicion of nonaccidental trauma.

    1. _____

    2. _____

    3. _____

    4. _____

    5. _____

21. (Circle the correct word.) The number of persons in the United States who are at or above retirement age is (increasing/decreasing).

22. List four strategies that will help to improve communication with patients who are hard of hearing.

    1. _____

    2. _____

    3. _____

    4. _____

23. A term that refers to a large group of disorders associated with brain damage or impaired cerebral function,

    particularly in the aged, is _____ .

24. *(Circle the correct phrase.)* Patients with Alzheimer disease or other conditions that affect mental function are more likely to lose their memory of (recent events/the distant past).

25. Demineralization, osteopenia, and osteoporosis are all terms that refer to the condition of aging that is

    characterized by _____ .

26. List three soft tissue changes that occur as a result of aging.

    1. _____

    2. _____

    3. _____

27. Open sores over bony prominences that occur when pressure on a limited area inhibits circulation are called

    _____ .

28. *(Circle the correct words.)* When adjusting exposure factors to compensate for osteopenia in the elderly, it is best to (increase/decrease) the (mA/kVp).

29. A degenerative inflammatory disease of the colon that is common in the elderly and is characterized by

    constipation and/or diarrhea with abdominal cramping is called _____ .

30. A degenerative condition of the nervous system that attacks the elderly and is characterized by fine tremors, a

    peculiar gait, and a lack of facial expression is called _____ .

Chapter 21

Image Critique

Exercise 1

Answer the following questions by selecting the best choice.

1. Image critique is the process that determines whether an image:
   1. is correctly identified.
   2. contains sufficient diagnostic quality.
   3. meets the minimum requirements of the request.
   A. 1 and 2
   B. 1 and 3
   C. 2 and 3
   D. 1, 2, and 3

2. Which of the following conditions should be observed when viewing radiographs?
   1. View each with a "hot light."
   2. Maintain clean view boxes.
   3. Maintain a low light level in the viewing area.
   A. 1 and 2
   B. 1 and 3
   C. 2 and 3
   D. 1, 2, and 3

3. When radiographs are viewed, the correct image orientation is:
   A. the way the image receptor (IR) was exposed.
   B. in the anatomic position.
   C. with the patient's right side toward the viewer's right side.
   D. dependent upon the institution's policy.

4. The term *esthetic quality* refers to the:
   A. eye appeal of the radiograph.
   B. position of the part on the IR.
   C. amount of detail in the image.
   D. amount of contrast in the image.

5. Images that lack esthetic quality may:
   1. show artifacts.
   2. be too dark or too light.
   3. display poor alignment of the body part.
   A. 1 and 2
   B. 1 and 3
   C. 2 and 3
   D. 1, 2, and 3

6. Which of the following would be a factor used to evaluate radiation safety?
   A. Contrast
   B. Density
   C. Collimation
   D. Patient positioning

7. (True/False) The decision to repeat a radiograph should be based on radiation safety.

8. (True/False) Keeping a log of repeated films aids the limited operator in evaluating problems and progressing toward esthetic quality.

9. Troubleshooting an image includes:
   1. deciding whether the film should be repeated.
   2. determining the cause of any problems.
   3. discussing the film with the patient's physician.
   A. 1 and 2
   B. 1 and 3
   C. 2 and 3
   D. 1, 2, and 3

10. (True/False) Radiographs with markings added after processing are not admissible in court.

11. (True/False) Errors in diagnosis can occur with incorrect position and exposure factors.

12. The factors that affect recorded detail include which of the following?
    1. Object-image distance
    2. Motion
    3. Screen speed
    A. 1 and 2
    B. 1 and 3
    C. 2 and 3
    D. 1, 2, and 3

13. Which of the following will decrease patient motion in the radiograph?
    A. Use of low-mA techniques
    B. Use of low-kVp techniques
    C. Provision of clear instructions
    D. Selection of a slow-speed screen if motion is anticipated

14. Film density problems can be caused by the:
    A. Bucky.
    B. processor.
    C. x-ray room temperature.
    D. darkroom temperature.

15. Anatomic structures may be excluded in the image because of:
    1. inaccurate collimation.
    2. improper IR size.
    3. improper selection of mA or kVp.

A. 1 and 2
B. 1 and 3
C. 2 and 3
D. 1, 2, and 3

16. Radiographs of fingers, hands, toes, and feet are positioned on the view box with the:
    A. distal aspects pointing up.
    B. distal aspects pointing down.

17. A limited operator would be repeating radiographs unnecessarily if his or her repeat rate exceeded:
    A. 1%.
    B. 4%.
    C. 10%.
    D. 15%.

18. Most experienced limited operators have a repeat rate of about:
    A. 1%.
    B. 4%.
    C. 10%.
    D. 15%.

Exercise 2

Answer the following questions.

1. What is the acronym that can help you remember how to accurately assess image quality?

   _____

2. What does each letter stand for in the acronym that answers question 1?

   Letter   **Definition**

   ____   _____

   ____   _____

   ____   _____

   ____   _____

   ____   _____

3. Describe the anatomic position.

   _____

   _____

_____

_____

_____

4. How often should view box bulbs be changed? Why?

_____

_____

_____

_____

Chapter 22

Ethics, Legal Considerations, and Professionalism

Answer the following questions.

1. List at least four characteristics that distinguish a profession from a nonprofessional occupation.

   1. _____

   2. _____

   3. _____

   4. _____

2. (True/False) Limited radiography is considered to be a profession.

3. (True/False) Professional attitudes and behaviors are expected of limited x-ray machine operators.

4. Define the following terms and give an example of each.

   1. Morals: _____

      _____

   2. Values: _____

      _____

   3. Ethics: _____

      _____

5. An aspirational document that establishes a high standard of professional conduct and assists the members of the radiologic technology profession in practicing ethical principles is the

   _____

6. Mandatory standards of minimally acceptable professional conduct for all registered radiologic technologists are contained in the document called the

   _____

   _____.

7. Write a brief phrase that characterizes the behavior prescribed in each principle of the Code of Ethics of the American Registry of Radiologic Technologists.

   Principle 1: _____

   Principle 2: _____

   Principle 3: _____

   Principle 4: _____

   Principle 5: _____

   Principle 6: _____

   Principle 7: _____

   Principle 8: _____

   Principle 9: _____

   Principle 10: _____

8. (True/False) The confidentiality of conversations between patients and limited operators is not protected by "legal privilege."

9. (True/False) It is ethical to discuss your patients with your friends as long as you don't mention the patients' names.

10. List the four basic steps involved in solving ethical dilemmas using the process of ethical analysis.

    1. _____

    2. _____

    3. _____

    4. _____

11. Using "A Patient's Bill of Rights" from this chapter, identify those patient rights for which a limited operator may have direct responsibility.

    _____

12. (True/False) Most procedures commonly performed by limited operators require that the patient sign an informed consent document.

13. (True/False) Parents, grandparents, or adult siblings may sign an informed consent form for a minor.

14. (True/False) Informed consent may be revoked by the patient at any time after signing.

15. Explain briefly why it is essential to maintain all credentials that are required for practice.

    _____

    _____

    _____

16. Match the types of intentional misconduct with their legal definitions.

   1. _____ Assault

   2. _____ Battery

   3. _____ False imprisonment

   4. _____ Invasion of privacy

   5. _____ Libel

   6. _____ Slander

   A. Unjustifiable detention

   B. Unlawful touching

   C. Written information that causes defamation of character

   D. Disclosure of confidential information

   E. Omission of reasonable care

   F. The threat of touching in an injurious way

   G. Verbal dissemination of information that causes loss of reputation

17. Failure to use reasonable care or caution is termed _____.

18. What is the standard of care that is used to legally define negligence?

   _____

19. The responsibility of health care providers for accountability in the area of patient confidentiality is legally

   prescribed in a federal law known by the acronym _____.

20. An act of negligence in the context of a professional relationship is defined as professional negligence or

   _____.

21. The employer is liable for employees' negligent acts that occur in the course of their work according to the legal

   doctrine of _____.

22. List three important steps you can take to reduce the likelihood of malpractice litigation.

   1. _____

   2. _____

   3. _____

23. Number the following list of human needs in order according to the hierarchy of needs, with 1 being the most basic level of needs and 6 being the highest level.

   _____ Love and acceptance

   _____ Nutrition and oxygen

   _____ Recognition

   _____ Recreation

   _____ Self-actualization

   _____ Safety

24. List good practices that represent responsible self-care by limited operators.

_____

_____

_____

_____

_____

25. List three positive actions for promoting teamwork and cooperation in the workplace.

    1. _____

    2. _____

    3. _____

26. Sensitivity to the needs of others that allows you to meet those needs constructively is called

    _____.

27. What is the best strategy for dealing with clinical situations in which you find it difficult to cope because the patient is vomiting or bleeding or acting inappropriately?

    _____

    _____

28. List reasons why limited operators should pursue continuing education, even if it is not required for the renewal of credentials.

    _____

    _____

    _____

    _____

29. List three nonverbal behaviors that enhance communication.

    1. _____

    2. _____

    3. _____

30. Explain what is meant by *validation of communication*.

    _____

    _____

    _____

31. List three useful strategies for successful communication under stress.

    1. _____

    2. _____

    3. _____

32. Write two questions other than those presented in the text that could be used to offer an adult patient a valid choice.

    1. _____

    2. _____

33. Match the following communication terms with the correct definitions.

    1. _____ Validation   A. Sensitivity to the needs of others

    2. _____ Aggression   B. Reaction to the distress of others

    3. _____ Empathy   C. Calm, firm expression of feelings or opinions

    4. _____ Assertion   D. Confirmation that a message is understood

    5. _____ Sympathy   E. Expression of angry or hostile feelings

                                             F. Disregard for the feelings of others

34. List signs or characteristics that might alert you to the fact that a patient is totally deaf.

    _____

    _____

    _____

    _____

35. List three ways in which the deaf may communicate.

    1. _____

    2. _____

    3. _____

36. (True/False) Patients who do not speak English are responsible for communicating effectively in a health care situation despite language barriers.

37. (True/False) When patients do not speak English, translation by a family member is preferable to translation by an interpreter who is not known by the patient.

38. (True/False) When using an interpreter you should talk directly to the patient as if the patient could understand you.

39. List common social practices in the United States that might be different in other cultures.

40. An old superstition of Mediterranean origin that is occasionally seen among Hispanic patients is called the *evil eye*, or *mal ojo*. This is a belief that _____.

41. Check the cultural groups listed below in which direct eye contact is generally acceptable.

    _____ The United States

    _____ Most Asian cultures

    _____ Native American cultures

    _____ Hispanic culture

    _____ Russian culture

42. Aggressive demands for service and attention by patients' families are most commonly a result of

    _____.

43. List three things you can do to support the anxious relatives of an injured patient.

    1. _____

    2. _____

    3. _____

44. A legal document that contains a record of the care and treatment received by a patient is called a

    _____.

45. Diagnostic images are owned by _____.

46. What should you do if a physician calls from across town and requests images that are in your files?

    _____

    _____

    _____

Chapter 23

Safety and Infection Control

Answer the following questions.

1. In the list below, check the three elements that must be present in order for a fire to burn.

   _____ Open flames

   _____ Fuel

   _____ Smoke

   _____ Oxygen

   _____ Electricity

   _____ Heat

2. (True/False) In case of an electric fire you should use a class A fire extinguisher or a water supply to put out the fire.

3. (True/False). Oxygen does not burn.

4. List three important fire safety precautions that should be observed when oxygen is in use.

   1. _____

   2. _____

   3. _____

5. What should you know about a clinical facility to be prepared in case of fire?

   _____

   _____

   _____

   _____

6. Give the acronym for remembering the four basic steps to take in case of fire. Write the meaning of each letter in the acronym.

   _____

   _____

   _____

   _____

7. Write the steps for safe use of a fire extinguisher as indicated by the acronym *PASS*.

   P: _____

   A: _____

   S: _____

   S: _____

8. Caution to avoid electric shock is especially important when using electricity around _____.

9. List steps that should be taken to provide safety in the case of a hazardous chemical spill, such as concentrated bleach or fixer solution.

   _____

   _____

   _____

   _____

10. The principles of proper body alignment, movement, and balance are referred to as _____

    _____.

11. *(Circle the correct phrase.)* When lifting a heavy object from the floor, you should (bend your body at the waist/bend at the hips and knees).

12. *(Circle the correct phrase.)* When moving a heavy object that is on wheels, you should (push it/pull it).

13. Label the names of the body positions shown in Fig. 23-1.

    A. _____

    B. _____

    C. _____

    D. _____

    E. _____

14. To relieve lumbosacral stress or abdominal strain when a patient is supine, a bolster is placed under the _____.

15. Inability to breathe when lying down is termed _____.

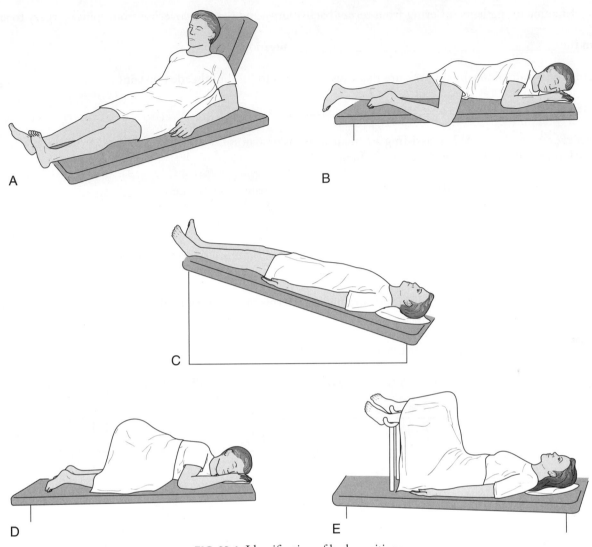

FIG. 23-1 Identification of body positions.

16. Check the positions below that are appropriate for nauseated patients to provide safety from possible aspiration of vomitus.

_____ Fowler

_____ Sims

_____ Trendelenburg

_____ Lateral recumbent

_____ Supine

17. Padding should be placed under bony prominences such as the sacrum, heels, or midthoracic curvature of older or

    debilitated patients for comfort and to prevent the development of _____.

18. When assisting a patient to lie down, place one arm _____ and the other

    _____.

19. It is preferable for patients suffering from recent back injuries and those recovering from spinal surgery to sit up

    from the _____ position.

20. A temporary state of low blood pressure that causes patients to feel lightheaded or faint when they first sit up is

    termed _____ .

21. *(Circle the correct phrase.)* When assisting a patient who has weakness on one side of the body to walk, position
    yourself on the patient's (strong side/weak side).

22. The most common type of fall associated with wheelchair transfer occurs when _____

    _____ .

23. (True/False) The use of sandbags to immobilize trembling extremities can assist in minimizing motion, even when
    the area of interest does not involve the extremity.

24. (True/False) The application of physical restraints to the arms or legs of an adult patient without the patient's
    consent requires a physician's order.

25. (True/False) An incident report must be completed only for occurrences that result in injury to a patient.

26. The four principal factors involved in the spread of disease, sometimes called the *cycle of infection*, are:

    1. _____

    2. _____

    3. _____

    4. _____

27. Match the following terms referring to microorganisms and other infectious agents with their definitions.

    1. _____ Normal flora

    2. _____ Pathogens

    3. _____ Bacteria

    4. _____ Viruses

    5. _____ Endospores

    6. _____ Fungi

    7. _____ Prions

    8. _____ Protozoa

    A. The smallest and least understood of all infectious agents

    B. Very small subcellular organisms such as those that cause influenza, chickenpox, and the common cold

    C. Bacterial forms that are resistant to heat, cold, and drying and can live without nourishment

    D. Agents that cause disease

    E. Complex single-cell animals that generally exist as free-living organisms

    F. Microorganisms that live on or within the body without causing disease

    G. Very small single-cell organisms with a cell wall and an atypical nucleus that lacks a membrane; named for their shapes, including bacilli, cocci, spirochetes, and spirilla

    H. Occur as single-celled yeast or as filament-like structures called molds

28. Describe the five indirect routes of disease transmission and give an example of each.

    1. Fomite: _____

       _____

    2. Vector: _____

       _____

    3. Vehicle: _____

       _____

    4. Airborne contamination: _____

       _____

    5. Droplet contamination: _____

       _____

29. The agency that monitors and studies the types of infections occurring in the nation and compiles and publishes

    statistical data about these infections is _____.

30. The infectious agent that causes acquired immunodeficiency syndrome (AIDS) is _____.

31. In the list below, check the types of contact that may result in the transmission of human immunodeficiency virus
    (HIV).

    _____ Shaking hands

    _____ Sexual intercourse

    _____ Eating of food prepared by an infected individual

    _____ Sharing of contaminated needles

    _____ Contact with drinking fountains

    _____ Contact with toilets

32. (True/False) There is no known cure for AIDS.

33. (True/False) The patient's right to confidentiality regarding AIDS diagnosis or HIV status may prevent you from
    being informed about the patient's status.

34. (True/False) There are thousands of documented, confirmed cases of HIV infection in health care workers
    resulting from accidental needle sticks.

35. The hepatitis B virus (HBV) is spread through contact with _____.

36. The types of hepatitis that are spread through contact with food or water contaminated with feces are type _____

    and type _____.

37. Vaccine is available to protect health care workers from infection by which hepatitis virus? _____

    _____.

38. If postexposure prophylaxis (PEP) is recommended following a needle stick injury, how soon after the injury

    should this therapy be administered? _____

39. Pulmonary tuberculosis is spread by means of _____

    _____

40. (True/False) Most of those who become infected with tubercle bacilli develop a clinical disease and become
    infectious to others.

41. (True/False) Lowered resistance because of immune deficiency, malnutrition, other illness, or old age may cause
    reactivation of a tuberculosis infection.

42. The simplest and most common method of testing for tuberculosis infection is the _____

    _____.

43. The Standard Precautions defined by the Centers for Disease Control and Prevention (CDC) call for the use of
    barriers whenever contact is anticipated with what four things?

    1. _____

    2. _____

    3. _____

    4. _____

44. List three pathogens that are commonly responsible for nosocomial infections.

    1. _____

    2. _____

    3. _____

45. The destruction of pathogens by chemical agents is called _____.

46. Treating items with heat, gas, or chemicals to make them germ free is called _____

    _____.

47. Decontamination of the hands using soap and water, an antiseptic hand wash, or an alcohol-based hand rub is
    called _____.

48. (True/False) Alcohol hand rubs are effective against most microorganisms.

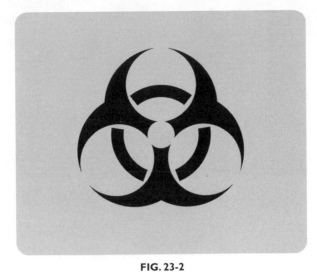

FIG. 23-2

49. (True/False) Hand hygiene is not necessary when gloves are worn.

50. When should washing with soap and water be used for hand hygiene instead of an alcohol rub? _____

    _____

51. As a cleaning agent for decontaminating environmental surfaces, the CDC recommends either a disinfectant registered by the Environmental Protection Agency as effective against HIV, HBV, and the tuberculosis

    bacterium or _____

52. Fig. 23-2 is a symbol that indicates _____.

53. (True/False) You should not remove anything from a hazardous waste container once it has been placed inside.

54. (True/False) To prevent needle stick injuries you should always recap needles.

55. A receptacle for the disposal of needles, syringes, and contaminated items capable of puncturing the skin is called a

    _____.

56. The quickest and most convenient means of sterilization for items that can withstand heat is

    _____.

57. The type of sterilization that is used for telephones, stethoscopes, blood pressure cuffs, and other equipment that

    cannot withstand heat is _____.

58. A germ-free area prepared for the use of sterile supplies and equipment is called a _____

    _____.

59. The first step in preparing a sterile field is to confirm the sterility of packaged supplies and equipment. List the criteria that indicate when packages are considered sterile.

    1. _____

    2. _____

    3. _____

60. *(Circle the correct phrase.)* When opening a sterile pack, open the first corner (toward you/away from you).

61. (True/False) It is all right to reach across a sterile field as long as you do not touch anything that is sterile.

62. (True/False) Any sterile object or field touched by an unsterile object or person becomes contaminated.

63. (True/False) Before adding a liquid to a sterile tray you should discard a small amount from the container to rinse the container's lip.

64. *(Circle the correct word.)* The (application/removal) of a dressing is a procedure that requires sterile technique.

Chapter 24

Assessing Patients and Managing Acute Situations

Answer the following questions.

1. List the three skills that will help you adequately determine patients' needs.

   1. _____

   2. _____

   3. _____

2. List steps you can take to reassure and comfort patients who feel anxious.

   _____

   _____

   _____

   _____

3. List considerations that might help meet patients' physiologic needs.

   _____

   _____

4. Loss of bladder control is termed _____.

5. List the six characteristics of a patient's chief complaint that should be addressed in the questions used to elicit a preliminary medical history of the complaint.

   1. _____

   2. _____

   3. _____

   4. _____

   5. _____

   6. _____

6. When a patient exhibits a bluish coloration in the mucous membranes of the lips and in the nail beds, the patient is said to be _____.

7. When a patient is described as diaphoretic, this means that the patient is _____.

8. Hot, dry skin may indicate that the patient has _____.

9. *(Circle the correct word.)* Rectal temperatures are (higher/lower) than oral temperatures.

10. *(Circle the correct word.)* Axillary temperatures are (higher/lower) than oral temperatures.

11. When is it *not* appropriate to take a patient's temperature orally?

_____

_____

12. A rapid pulse, when the heart beats more than 100 times per minute, is called _____.

13. A pulse that is described as thready is one that is both _____ and _____.

14. *(Circle the correct word.)* The first or upper number in a blood pressure value is the (diastolic/systolic) pressure.

15. *(Circle the correct word.)* The term *hypertension* refers to (high/low) blood pressure.

16. The cuff and gauge for measuring blood pressure is called a(n):

    A. stethoscope.

    B. sphygmomanometer.

    C. tympanic thermometer.

    D. aneroid barometer.

17. List two steps you should take to ensure that emergency supplies are ready for use when an emergency arises.

    1. _____

    2. _____

18. *(Circle the correct term.)* In an emergency situation, oxygen is usually administered by means of a (mask/nasal cannula).

19. The usual flow rate for oxygen administration by face mask is _____.

20. *(Circle the correct word.)* Patients suffering from emphysema should receive an oxygen flow rate that is (greater/less) than the usual or average rate.

21. When a patient is unable to swallow or to cope with secretions, blood, or vomitus, you should prepare to assist with _____.

22. If a patient complains of sudden, intense pain under the sternum, you should assume until proven otherwise that the patient might be having _____.

23. When a patient suddenly loses consciousness, the first thing you should do is _____.

24. Lack of effective circulation to the central nervous system for 5 minutes can cause _____.

25. A rapid, weak, and ineffective heartbeat caused by interruption of the electric signals that control the

    heart is called _____.

26. When bleeding or swelling occurs inside the skull, seizures, loss of consciousness, or respiratory arrest may occur

    because of increased _____.

27. When a blow to the head causes damage on the side of the head opposite the side of the blow, this is termed a

    _____.

28. List the four levels of consciousness.

    1. _____

    2. _____

    3. _____

    4. _____

29. A fracture in which the bone protrudes through the skin is called a _____

30. Continuous, abnormal blood flow is called _____.

31. Redness of the skin is termed _____.

32. A severe allergic reaction is termed _____ or _____.

33. An antihistamine medication, such as diphenhydramine, may be given as a treatment for _____.

34. Anaphylaxis is a type of shock caused by _____.

35. An individual who is terribly thirsty, urinates copious amounts frequently, and has fruity-smelling breath may be

    approaching a state of _____.

36. An enzyme normally produced in the pancreas that aids in the digestion of glucose is _____.

37. A cerebrovascular accident (CVA) is also called a _____.

38. List the warning signs of CVA.

    1. _____

    2. _____

    3. _____

    4. _____

5. _____

6. _____

39. A transient ischemic attach is a mild, temporary form of a _____.

40. In the event of a seizure, your first duty is to _____.

41. A brief loss of consciousness (absence) during which the patient stares or may lose balance and fall is a

type of _____.

42. When an anxious patient hyperventilates and complains of feeling faint or dizzy, what should you do?

_____.

_____.

43. *Syncope* is another term for _____.

44. A sensation of dizziness in which the patient feels as if the room is moving or whirling is termed _____.

45. Squeezing firmly against the nasal septum for 10 minutes is a treatment for _____.

Chapter 25

Medications and Their Administration

Answer the following questions.

1. List duties related to medication administration that a limited operator may perform, even if not permitted to actually administer the medication.

   1. _____

   2. _____

   3. _____

   4. _____

   5. _____

2. Whose duty is it to determine the route of administration for a medication? _____

3. (True/False) A standing order might allow a nurse to administer a specific dose of nitroglycerin to a patient experiencing angina when the physician is not present.

4. (True/False) Checking expiration dates on medication supplies is not important in physicians' offices and clinics because such supplies are used infrequently.

5. The name of a drug that identifies its specific chemical composition is called its _____.

6. The brand name given to a product by its manufacturer is called its _____ or _____ name.

7. Match the following types of medication effects with their definitions.

   1. _____ Toxic   A. Produces a specific action that promotes a desired effect

   2. _____ Agonistic   B. Causes an unusual or peculiar effect, or the opposite of the expected effect

   3. _____ Antagonistic   C. Term for drugs whose combined effect is beyond the individual effects of each

   4. _____ Synergistic   D. Has poisonous consequences

   5. _____ Idiosyncratic   E. Prevents or reverses the effects of other drugs

8. The government agency that sets standards for control of drugs is the _____.

9. The efficacy of a drug refers to its _____.

10. The potency of a drug refers to its _____.

11. Match the following routes of administration with their definitions.

1. _____ Topical	A. Inside the cheek
2. _____ Intradermal	B. Under the skin
3. _____ Intramuscular	C. Between the skin layers
4. _____ Sublingual	D. Within a vein
5. _____ Buccal	E. Under the tongue
6. _____ Subcutaneous	F. Within the muscle
7. _____ Intravenous	G. By mouth, swallowed
8. _____ Oral	H. On the skin

12. Match the following drug classes with their applications. The applications may be used more than once.

1. _____ Antihistamine	A. Antimicrobial, prevents or treats infection
2. _____ Antibiotic	B. Antiinflammatory, treats inflammation, including that caused by allergic reactions
3. _____ NSAID	C. Tranquilizer, sedates
4. _____ Disinfectant	D. Analgesic, relieves pain
5. _____ Corticosteroid	E. Antiallergic, relieves symptoms of allergic reactions
6. _____ Benzodiazepine	F. Anesthetic, eliminates sensation

13. Medication effect is determined to some degree by the water content of body tissues, which is termed _____ _____.

14. Match the following terms related to pharmacokinetics with their definitions.

1. _____ Excretion	A. The process by which the body transforms drugs into an inactive form that can be eliminated from the body
2. _____ Absorption	B. The process by which the drug enters the systemic circulation to provide a desired effect
3. _____ Metabolism	C. The elimination of drugs from the body
4. _____ Distribution	D. The means by which drugs travel to the site of action

15. The most common mechanism of drug action is the binding of drugs to _____.

16. Drugs are administered to produce a predictable physiologic response called the _____.

17. Opioids and other substances whose availability is strictly regulated or outlawed because of their potential for abuse or addiction are called _____ substances.

18. Life-threatening respiratory depression is a possible side effect following the administration of

_____.

19. A specific drug that treats a toxic effect is called a(an) _____.

20. If a child weighs 30 lb, what is the child's weight in kilograms? _____

21. If a drug is supplied in a strength of 5 mg/ml, and you want to administer 15 mg, you will need _____ ml.

22. If 5 ml of a drug has been administered and the strength is 30 mcg/ml, what dose was given? _____

23. (True/False) The Occupational Safety and Health Administration regulations now require the use of engineering controls to decrease the risk to health care workers from contaminated needle sticks.

24. (True/False) A 22-gauge needle is larger around than a 18-gauge needle and delivers a given volume of fluid more rapidly.

25. For intramuscular injection in small children, the preferred muscle site is the _____.

26. The height of the bottle or bag used for intravenous infusion affects the flow rate and should always be _____ inches above the level of the vein.

27. When the area around an intravenous infusion injection site is cool, swollen, and boggy, these are signs that

_____.

28. When extravasation occurs during an intravenous injection or infusion, you should _____ _____.

29. (True/False) You should wear protective gloves when giving injections.

30. (True/False) Aseptic technique should always be followed for injection procedures.

31. List the information that must be included when the administration of a medication is charted.

_____

_____

_____

Chapter 26

Medical Laboratory Skills

Answer the following questions.

1. Standard Precautions were developed to protect health care workers from infection with

   _____

2. The essence of Standard Precautions is embodied in the statement that

   _____

3. List the three essential aspects of Standard Precautions as they relate to handling blood and urine.

   1. _____

   2. _____

   3. _____

4. Any refuse that is poisonous or dangerous to living creatures is termed

   _____

5. Objects that can puncture the skin such as needles, glass tubes, glass slides, and finger lancets must be disposed of

   in a _____

6. The technique of entering a vein with a needle to withdraw a blood sample is termed

   _____

7. The veins most commonly used for obtaining blood samples are located in the

   _____

8. The evacuated plastic tubes used for blood specimen collection have color-coded stoppers that indicate

   _____

9. List two ways in which the handling of blood specimen tubes that have additives differs from the handling of those that do not.

   1. _____

   2. _____

10. (True/False) An evacuated blood specimen tube cannot be used a second time following an unsuccessful venipuncture.

11. State the needle gauge and length for routine venipuncture:

    _____ gauge, _____ inches in length.

12. A standard venipuncture needle is actually two needles attached to a threaded plastic hub. The needle mounted

    to the threaded side of the hub is designed to puncture _____. The other needle,

    mounted to the nonthreaded end of the hub, is for puncturing _____.

13. (True/False) Special venipuncture needles with engineered sharps injury protection are available to minimize the risk of needle stick injury to personnel and to comply with the requirements of the Occupational Safety and Health Administration.

14. (True/False) Venipuncture needle holders (barrels) are reusable items.

15. A tight band placed around the arm to facilitate distention of the vein for venipuncture is called a

    _____.

16. Alcohol prep wipes are generally used to cleanse the skin for venipuncture, but povidone-iodine wipes must be

    used if the specimen is to being collected for _____ or

    _____.

17. (True/False) Some manufacturers produce evacuated tubes with stoppers covered by plastic caps to minimize aerosol production; these caps eliminate the need to use a shield when opening specimen tubes.

18. List three sites that should be avoided when selecting a site for venipuncture.

    1. _____

    2. _____

    3. _____

19. Choice of a vein for venipuncture is based on _____.

20. *(Circle the correct word.)* When obtaining a blood specimen, you should engage the vacuum tube on the internal needle (before/after) the external needle is properly situated in the vein.

21. *(Circle the correct word.)* When all blood specimens have been obtained, you should remove the last tube from the needle holder (before/after) removing the needle from the vein.

22. Failure of the tube to fill with blood during venipuncture means that

    _____.

23. The physical, microscopic, and/or chemical examination of urine is termed _____.

24. List the three components of a routine urinalysis.

    1. _____

    2. _____

    3. _____

25. What should you do to maintain the quality and accuracy of reagent strips?

    _____

    _____

26. (True/False) *Urinalysis tube* is another term for a urine specimen collection cup.

27. When should a urine specimen be collected to obtain the greatest amount of diagnostic information?

    _____

28. Urine collected regardless of the time of day is termed a _____

    _____.

29. The correct method for collecting a urine specimen is called the _____

    _____.

30. *(Circle the correct phrase.)* When a female cleanses the labia for a clean-catch midstream specimen, the cleansing sponge or towelette is wiped in a(n) (anterior to posterior/posterior to anterior) direction.

31. If a urine specimen cannot be analyzed promptly, how should the specimen be handled when first obtained and before analysis?

    _____

    _____

    _____

32. List the two characteristics to be assessed in a macroscopic (visual) examination of urine.

    1. _____

    2. _____

33. (True/False) When a urine reagent strip is read, timing is critical, and the test result must be read in the time indicated by the manufacturer.

34. When the color of a urine reagent strip does not match any of the reference colors and the test has been repeated with the same results using a strip from a different bottle, what should you do?

    _____

35. When multiple end-point colors are noted within the test area for blood, revealing a green speckled pattern overlying an orange background, the result is reported as

    _____.

36. If it is necessary to perform a urinalysis during the menstrual period, what method is used to prevent contamination of the specimen with menstrual blood?

    _____

    _____

37. List the abnormal results from analyses of the chemical and physical characteristics of urine that indicate the need for a microscopic examination of the urine sediment.

    _____

38. A special electric device in laboratories that spins the urine tubes rapidly to separate solids from liquid for the microscopic evaluation of sediment is called a _____.

Chapter 27

Additional Procedures for Assessment and Diagnosis

Answer the following questions.

1. What should be the setting of a balance scale before the patient steps on it to be weighed?

   _____

   _____

2. *(Circle the correct word.)* When a patient is weighed on a balance scale, the weight on the (upper/lower) calibration bar should be adjusted first.

3. When a patient is standing on a balance scale and the scale is in balance, how is the patient's weight determined?

   _____

   _____

4. When a digital electronic scale is used, if the weight readout keeps changing or does not appear promptly, this is

   most likely an indication that _____.

5. *(Circle the correct word.)* When the height of a patient is measured using the calibration rod of a balance scale, the rod should be raised and the measuring bar unfolded into the horizontal position (before/after) the patient steps onto the platform.

6. A patient's weight should be recorded to the nearest

   _____.

7. A patient's height should be recorded to the nearest

   _____.

8. Define the following conditions, which can be identified by simple vision screening tests.

   1. Myopia: _____

   2. Hyperopia: _____

   3. Presbyopia: _____

9. For children who have not learned the alphabet or patients who are unfamiliar with the English alphabet, distance

   vision is tested using the _____ chart.

10. Distance vision assessment is usually made at a distance of _____.

11. Write the abbreviations for the following terms used to chart the results of vision tests.

    Right eye: _____

    Left eye: _____

12. The classic method of evaluating color perception is the _____ test.

13. A graphic representation of tiny electric currents generated within the heart is a diagnostic tool used to assess heart

    disease and is called a(n) _____.

14. Label the waves that represent a complete cardiac cycle in the electrocardiogram (ECG) tracing in Fig. 27-1.

    1. _____

    2. _____

    3. _____

    4. _____

    5. _____

    6. _____

    7. _____

    8. _____

    9. _____

    10. _____

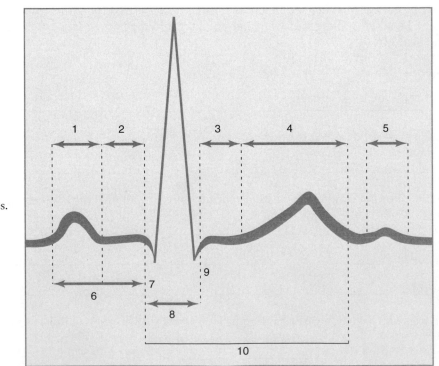

FIG. 27-1 ECG waves.

15. List the three types of leads that are used in a routine diagnostic ECG study. In each of the three categories, state the abbreviation or designation of each specific lead.

    1. _____

    2. _____

    3. _____

16. What aspect of the recording is controlled by the standard (STD) settings on an ECG machine?

    _____

17. If the amplitude of the QRS complex on an ECG is so great that it causes the stylus to move off the paper, what should you do?

    _____

18. The speed of the paper feed must be standardized for the tracing to be interpreted accurately. The universal

    recording speed is _____.

19. *(Circle the correct phrase.)* When connecting the patient cable to the electrodes, each lead wire (may be connected to any electrode/must be connected to a specific electrode.)

20. Match the features and artifacts on the following ECG tracings with their descriptions.

    1. _____

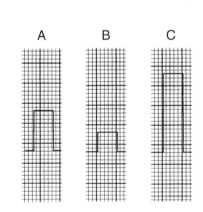

A. Subtle wandering baseline
B. Lead codes
C. Interrupted baseline
D. Standardization marks
E. Alternating current artifact
F. Major wandering baseline
G. Muscle artifact

    2. _____

    Marking Code

    .
    . .
    . . .
    –
    – –
    – – –
    – .
    – . .
    – . . .
    – . . . .
    – . . . . .
    – . . . . . .

3. _____

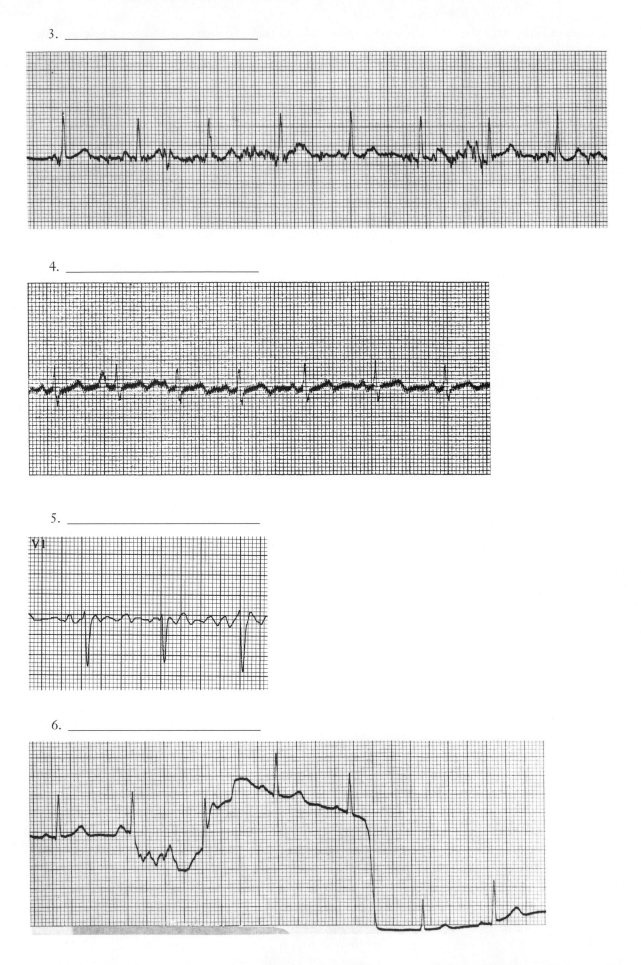

4. _____

5. _____

6. _____

7. _____

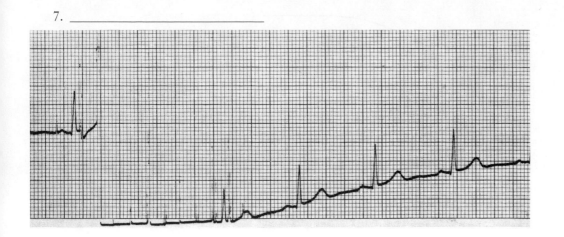

21. What type of compound is used to enhance the electric contact between ECG electrodes and the patient's skin?

_____.

22. (True/False) When the electrodes are all connected in preparation for an ECG, you should arrange the cords so that they lie on the patient's body.

23. Recording of ECG tracings during strenuous exercise is called a(n) _____

_____.

24. The measurement of lung airflow using a special machine is called _____.

25. List the two basic types of spirometers.

1. _____

2. _____

26. Identify the two types of spirometric graphs in the following illustrations.

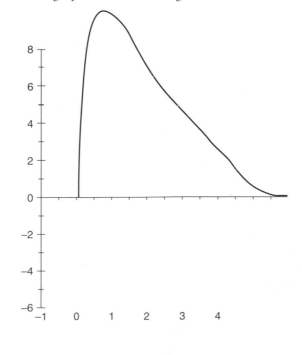

    1. _____

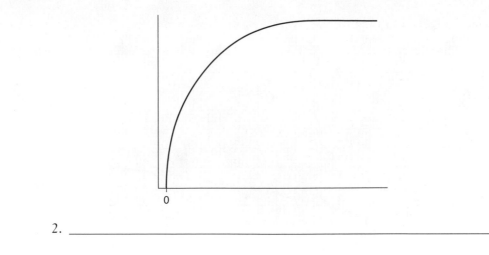

0

2. _____

27. List the three characteristics of a satisfactory forced expiration maneuver.

1. _____

2. _____

3. _____

28. How many satisfactory forced expiration graphs constitute a complete test?

_____

29. What is the maximum number of attempts that should be made to obtain the required number of satisfactory forced expiration graphs?

_____

30. List five contraindications for forced expiration spirometry.

1. _____

2. _____

3. _____

4. _____

5. _____

Chapter 28

Bone Densitometry

Exercise 1

Answer the following questions by selecting the best choice.

1. The abbreviation *DXA* stands for:
   A. double energy x-ray absorptiometry.
   B. double energy x-ray attenuation.
   C. dual energy x-ray absorptiometry.
   D. dual energy x-ray attenuation.

2. The most common sites scanned in bone densitometry are the:
   A. lumbar spine, forearm.
   B. lumbar spine, os calcis.
   C. forearm, proximal femur.
   D. lumbar spine, proximal femur.

3. What would be the most common preparation for DXA scanning?
   A. Nothing by mouth for 4 hours prior
   B. No dairy products for 24 hours prior
   C. 32 oz of water 6 hours prior
   D. No calcium tablets for 24 hours prior

4. Radiation exposure for a typical DXA scan is:
   A. 1 to 5 mrem.
   B. 1 to 5 rem.
   C. 200 to 400 mrem.
   D. 200 to 400 rem.

5. The T-score involves a direct comparison with:
   A. a young adult population.
   B. an age-matched (peer) population.
   C. a female population.
   D. a male population.

6. The Z-score involves a direct comparison with:
   A. a young adult population.
   B. an age-matched (peer) population.
   C. a female population.
   D. a male population.

7. Bone mineral density (BMD) is calculated as:
   A. BMC × area.
   B. BMC/area.
   C. area/BMC.
   D. area × BMC.

8. Reproducibility of DXA scan results is directly related to:
   A. the patient's pharmacologic treatment.
   B. the technologist's positioning techniques.
   C. the patient's calcium and vitamin D intake.
   D. the type of equipment used.

9. The gold standard technique in diagnostic testing for osteoporosis is:
   A. quantitative ultrasound (QUS).
   B. central table scanning (DXA).
   C. heel scanning (x-ray).
   D. general x-ray.

10. Baseline positioning is critical:
    A. because all follow-up scans are compared with the baseline scan.
    B. for accurate monitoring of change over time.
    C. because it is the most accurate or true measure of BMD.
    D. all of the above.

Exercise 2

Answer the following questions.

1. Describe the process of bone remodeling and its two main components.

    _____

    _____

    _____

2. Where is the x-ray tube in a DXA machine?

    _____

3. Describe the subtraction method used in BMD calculation.

    _____

    _____

    _____

    _____

4. Name the three types of beam utilized in DXA.

    _____

    _____

    _____

5. What is the formula for calculating BMD?

    _____

6. Name two contraindications to performing a DXA scan.

    _____

    _____

7. Describe the difference between accuracy and precision in bone densitometry.

    _____

    _____

8. List the three primary considerations when practicing proper radiation protection in DXA scanning.

    1. _____

    2. _____

    3. _____

9. What is the minimal distance a DXA operator should be from the x-ray source of a DXA machine?

_____

10. Define the difference between primary and secondary osteoporosis.

_____

_____

_____

_____

11. What are the most common skeletal sites scanned when DXA is performed?

_____

12. What is the correct procedure to follow after any bone assessment equipment has failed a quality assurance test?

_____

_____

_____

_____

_____

Exercise 3

Match the following terms with their definitions or descriptions.

1. _____ Weight bearing	A. Region of interest
2. _____ NOF	B. World Health Organization
3. _____ Precision	C. Postmenopausal or age-related osteoporosis
4. _____ PA lumbar spine	D. Standard deviation
5. _____ WHO	E. Percent coefficient of variation
6. _____ SD	F. Disease- or medication-induced osteoporosis
7. _____ %CV	G. Reached at about age 30 to 35
8. _____ Mean	H. Exercise that works against gravity
9. _____ 1200 mg	I. Daily recommended amount of vitamin D for patients over 50
10. _____ Secondary osteoporosis	J. Compares BMD with values for an age-matched group
11. _____ ROI	K. Measure of x-ray voltage
12. _____ 33%	L. Average
13. _____ AP lumbar spine	M. Projection of the lumbar spine in the DXA image
14. _____ Accuracy	N. Daily recommended amount of calcium for patients over 50
15. _____ Serial scans	O. Position of the patient for the lumbar spine DXA scan
16. _____ T-score	P. Relates to the stability of the DXA system
17. _____ Z-score	Q. Method of saving electronic patient data
18. _____ Primary osteoporosis	R. Bone mineral content
19. _____ 800 to 1000 IU	S. Preferred ROI for the forearm DXA scan
20. _____ kVp	T. Measure of absorbed dose of radiation

21. _____ mA
22. _____ Archive
23. _____ Peak bone mass
24. _____ BMC
25. _____ Gray

U. National Osteoporosis Foundation
V. Relates to the technologist's ability to reproduce the same positioning
W. Compares BMD with values for normal young adults
X. Measure of the rate of current flow in an x-ray tube
Y. DXA scans performed after the baseline scans

Exercise 4

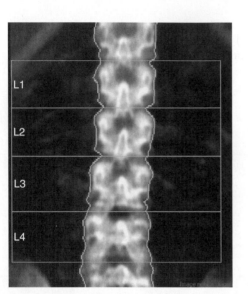

FIG. 28-1 Lumbar spine. (Courtesy Erickson Retirement Bone Health Program, 2008.)

1. (Yes/No) Was the lumbar spine scan in Figure 28-1 acquired correctly?

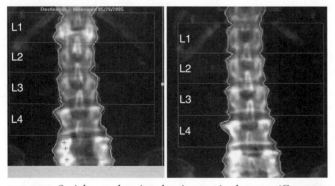

FIG. 28-2 Serial scan showing densitometric changes. (Courtesy Erickson Retirement Bone Health Program, 2008.)

2. The serial lumbar spine scan in Figure 28-2 shows densitometric changes.

A. Indicate the change that has occurred and explain how it will affect the analysis of the lumbar spine scan.

_____

_____

_____

B. Describe the steps the technologist must take to ensure proper comparison with the baseline lumbar spine scan.

_____

_____

_____

_____

_____

_____

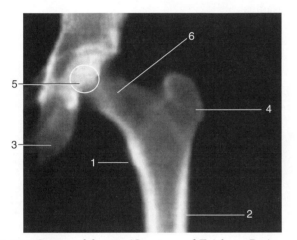

FIG. 28-3 Image of femur. (Courtesy of Erickson Retirement Bone Health Program, 2008.)

3. Match the anatomical parts listed below with the corresponding numbers in the accompanying image of the proximal femur.

   Greater trochanter _____

   Femoral neck _____

   Femoral head _____

   Pelvic ischium _____

   Lesser trochanter _____

   Femoral shaft _____

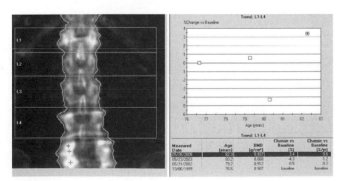

FIG. 28-4 Image of lumbar spine and baseline scan data. (Courtesy of Erickson Retirement Bone Health Program, 2008.)

4. Examine the lumbar spine image in Figure 28-4. What can you tell has happened to cause such an increase from the baseline scan values?

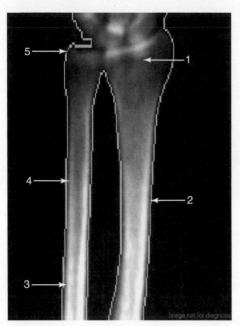

FIG. 28-5 Image of the forearm. (Courtesy of Erickson Retirement Bone Health Program, 2008.)

5. Match the anatomical parts listed below with the corresponding numbers in the accompanying image of the forearm.

Ulna _____

Radius _____

Distal radius _____

Proximal ulna _____

Ulnar styloid _____

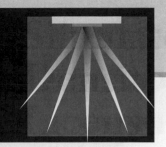

Section II

Preparation Guide for the American Registry of Radiologic Technologists Examination for the Limited Scope of Practice in Radiography

Introduction

This guide is provided to help you prepare to successfully complete the licensure examination for the limited scope of practice area in which you are or will be working. We have included helpful suggestions for optimizing your study time and a simulated examination to help you identify your areas of strength and weakness. All suggestions and discussions are based on the American Registry of Radiologic Technologists (ARRT) Content Specifications for the Examination for the Limited Scope of Practice in Radiography. We have done this for two reasons: first, this is a comprehensive examination covering all relevant areas of practice; and second, it is likely that the licensure agency in your state uses this examination. If your state does not use this examination you will still be well prepared if you use the ARRT Content Specifications as your study guide. For your convenience, we have included the most recent ARRT Content Specifications in this guide.

If you are using *Radiography Essentials for Limited Practice* and this accompanying Workbook, it is likely that you are participating in an educational program designed to prepare you both to work in a given practice area and to successfully pass the appropriate state licensure examination. This guide should assist you in both these endeavors. Completing the simulated examination will help you identify knowledge that you have already acquired and knowledge that you have yet to master. Since the simulated examination was constructed to assess content identified in the ARRT Content Specifications, it is appropriate to provide an overview of the latter document before moving on to the examination.

The ARRT Content Specifications for the Examination for the Limited Scope of Practice in Radiography covers five practice areas. These include chest, extremities, skull/sinuses, spine, and podiatry. The Content Specifications indicate that there are two components to each practice area licensure examination: a core module that everyone completes, and one or more radiographic procedures modules. The core module assesses knowledge in the areas of radiation protection, equipment operation, image production and evaluation, and patient care. According to the Content Specification document, the ARRT believes that all individuals licensed in limited scope radiography should know this information. Which of the radiographic procedures modules you take will depend on your area of practice. If your practice area is limited to chest radiography, you will complete only the chest module. However, if there is a licensure category in your state that allows radiography in all the procedural areas, you will complete all five modules. Licensure laws differ by state, and each licensure agency has its own procedures and guidelines.

The most valuable component of the Content Specifications is the outline of each content area covered on the examination. The numbers in parentheses in this outline indicate how many questions on the examination assess some aspect of knowledge in the designated area. The value to you is that this information will help you determine how much time and effort to spend on certain topics. Without using this information as a guide, you may waste valuable time learning information that is not included on the examination. However, we are not suggesting that you deviate from the curriculum established by your state agency or by your teacher. This guide is to help you prepare for the state licensure examination, not to prepare you to work in your practice area. You will need skills that cannot be directly assessed by a written examination.

The limited scope simulated examination is located after the ARRT Content Specifications in this section. You will find a core module and five radiographic procedures modules. You should complete the core module portion of the examination, regardless of your practice area. After completing the core module, complete the module or modules appropriate for your practice area. You should schedule time to complete all relevant portions of the examination at the same time. This will give you experience completing an examination of that length and give you some idea of how long it will take you to do so.

The core module consists of 100 questions, as prescribed in the ARRT Content Specifications, and contains the appropriate number of questions from each of the four content areas: radiation protection (35), equipment operation and quality control (12), image production and evaluation (38), and patient care and education (15). The questions are further focused to cover content specified in the outline for each content area. You will see that there are more content topics in each outline than there are questions included in the examination. This means that some content will not be assessed with a question, both on the simulated examination and on your actual state licensure examination. That is why it is important for you to review all topics included in each content outline in the ARRT Content Specifications. You cannot rely only on the simulated examination to prepare you for your state licensure examination.

The five radiographic procedures modules are located after the core module. Each contains the appropriate number of questions prescribed in the ARRT Content Specifications for the five modules: chest (20), extremities (25), skull/sinuses (20), spine (25), and podiatric radiography (20). The questions are further focused to cover content specified in the outline for each module. As mentioned in the previous paragraph, there are more content topics in each outline than there are questions included in the examination. Therefore, some content will not be assessed with a question, both on the simulated examination and on your actual state licensure examination. For this reason, you should review all topics included in each content outline in the ARRT Content Specifications.

The answers to all simulated examination questions in each examination module are located after the last question in the module. We have included the correct answer (ANS), as well as the textbook chapter in *Radiography Essentials for Limited Practice* in which the information is located (REF), the designator for the ARRT Content Specifications topic outline item (OBJ) that the question is designed to assess, and the topic (TOP) addressed by the question. This information will allow you to easily find and review text material that you have not yet mastered.

Your timeline to prepare for the state licensure examination should be something like the following:

- Participate in the educational program.
- Complete all workbook exercises related to the given area of practice. Don't waste time on radiographic procedures chapters outside your licensure area. This activity is especially important if you are not in a formal education program.
- Complete the simulated examination.
- Analyze the results of your examination to identify information you have not yet mastered.
- Review information related to questions you missed on the examination. It may be helpful to repeat relevant workbook exercises.
- Complete the simulated examination again and analyze the results. Review additional information, as needed.
- Successfully complete the state limited scope licensure examination!

ARRT Content Specifications for the Examination for the Limited Scope of Practice in Radiography

CONTENT SPECIFICATIONS FOR THE EXAMINATION FOR THE LIMITED SCOPE OF PRACTICE IN RADIOGRAPHY

Content Specifications Effective with the January 2009 Examination

The purpose of the American Registry of Radiologic Technologists examination for the Limited Scope of Practice in Radiography is to assess the knowledge and cognitive skills required to radiograph selected anatomic regions (chest, extremities, etc.). These content specifications represent a subset of the content specifications that were developed for general radiography through the ARRT Practice Analysis Project. The ARRT administers the examination at a state's request under contractual arrangement and provides the results directly to the state. This examination is not associated with any type of certification by the ARRT.

It is the philosophy of the ARRT that an individual licensed in limited scope radiography possess the same knowledge and cognitive skill, *in his or her specific area of radiography*, as general radiographers. For example, if an individual is licensed to take radiographs only of the spine, then that individual should be as knowledgeable about the spine as the general radiographer. However, that individual is not expected to demonstrate knowledge of radiographic procedures related to other anatomic regions (e.g., skull, chest). All individuals licensed in limited scope radiography are required to demonstrate fundamental knowledge and cognitive skill in the basic areas of radiation protection, equipment operation, image production and evaluation, and patient care.

The modules covered by the examination are outlined below. Subsequent pages describe in detail the topics covered within each module. All candidates take the CORE module of the examination and one or more RADIOGRAPHIC PROCEDURE modules, depending on the type of license for which they have applied.

Core Module		Number of Questions	Testing Time
A.	Radiation Protection	35	
B.	Equipment Operation and Quality Control	12	
C.	Image Production and Evaluation	38	
D.	Patient Care and Education	15	
	Total for Core Module	100	1 hr, 40 min
Radiographic Procedure Modules			
E.1	Chest	20	20 min
E.2	Extremities	25	25 min
E.3	Skull/Sinuses	20	20 min
E.4	Spine	25	25 min
E.5	Podiatric Radiography	20*	25 min

*The podiatry section may include 1 or 2 additional unscored (pilot) questions.

A. RADIATION PROTECTION (35)

I. Biological Aspects of Radiation (7)

A. Radiosensitivity

  1. dose-response relationships

  2. relative tissue radio sensitivities (e.g., LET, RBE)

  3. cell survival and recovery (LD_{50})

B. Somatic Effects

  1. short-term versus long-term effects

  2. acute vs. chronic effects

  3. carcinogenesis

  4. eye/thyroid

  5. reproductive (sterility)

C. Systemic Responses

  1. CNS

  2. hemopoietic

  3. skin

  4. GI

D. Embryonic and Fetal Risks

E. Genetic Impact

  1. genetic significant dose

  2. goals of gonadal shielding

II. Minimizing Patient Exposure (12)

A. Exposure Factors

  1. kVp

  2. mAs

B. Shielding

  1. rationale for use

  2. types

  3. placement

C. Beam Restriction

  1. purpose of primary beam restriction

  2. types (e.g., collimators)

D. Filtration

  1. effect on skin and organ exposure

  2. effect on average beam energy

  3. NCRP recommendations (NCRP #102, minimum filtration in useful beam)

E. Exposure Reduction

  1. patient positioning

  2. patient communication

F. Image Receptors (e.g., types, relative speed, digital vs. film)

A. RADIATION PROTECTION (cont.)

III.   Personnel Protection (8)

    A.   Sources of Radiation Exposure

        1.   primary x-ray beam

        2.   secondary radiation

            a.   scatter

            b.   leakage

        3.   patient as source

    B.   Basic Methods of Protection

        1.   time

        2.   distance

        3.   shielding

    C.   Protective Devices

        1.   types

        2.   attenuation properties

        3.   minimum lead equivalent (NCRP #102)

IV.   Radiation Exposure and Monitoring (8)

    A.   Units of Measurement[*]

        1.   absorbed dose (rad)

        2.   dose equivalent (rem)

        3.   exposure (Roentgen)

    B.   Dosimeters

        1.   types

        2.   proper use

    C.   NCRP Recommendations for Personnel Monitoring (NCRP #116)

        1.   occupational exposure

        2.   public exposure

        3.   embryo/fetus exposure

        4.   ALARA and dose equivalent limits

        5.   evaluation and maintenance of personnel dosimetry records

---

[*]Conventional units are generally used. However, questions referenced to specific reports (e.g., NCRP) will use SI units to be consistent with such reports.

B. EQUIPMENT OPERATION AND QUALITY CONTROL (12)

I. Principles of Radiation Physics (4)

A. X-Ray Production

1. source of free electrons (e.g., thermionic emission)

2. acceleration of electrons

3. focusing of electrons

4. deceleration of electrons

B. Target Interactions

1. bremsstrahlung

2. characteristic

C. X-Ray Beam

1. frequency and wavelength

2. beam characteristics

   a. quality

   b. quantity

   c. primary vs. remnant (exit)

3. inverse square law

4. fundamental properties (e.g., travel in straight lines, ionize matter)

D. Photon Interactions with Matter

1. Compton effect

2. photoelectric absorption

3. coherent (classical) scatter

4. attenuation by various tissues

   a. thickness of body part (density)

   b. type of tissue (atomic number)

II. Radiographic Equipment (4)

A. Components of Basic Radiographic Unit

1. operating console

2. x-ray tube construction

   a. electron sources

   b. target materials

   c. induction motor

3. manual exposure controls

4. beam restriction devices

B. X-Ray Generator, Transformers, and Rectification System

1. basic principles

2. phase, pulse, and frequency

C. Image Display

1. viewing conditions (i.e., luminance, ambient lighting)

2. spatial resolution

3. contrast resolution or dynamic range

4. DICOM gray scale function

5. window level and window width

D. Image Acquisition and Readout (e.g., PSP photo-stimulable phosphor)

III. Quality Control of Radiographic Equipment and Accessories (4)

A. Beam Restriction

1. light field to radiation field alignment

2. central ray alignment

B. Recognition of Malfunctions

C. Digital and Film-screen Image Receptor Systems

1. artifacts (e.g., non-uniformity, erasure)

2. maintenance (e.g., detector fog)

D. Shielding Accessories (e.g., lead apron testing)

C. IMAGE PRODUCTION AND EVALUATION (38)

I. Selection of Technical Factors (30)

   A. Factors Affecting Radiographic Quality. Refer to Attachment D to clarify terms that may occur on the exam. (X indicates topics covered on the examination)

	1. Density*	2. Contrast	3. Recorded Detail	4. Distortion
a. mAs	X			
b. kVp	X	X		
c. OID		X (air gap)	X	X
d. SID	X		X	X
e. focal spot size			X	
f. filtration	X	X		
g. film-screen combinations	X		X	
h. beam restriction	X	X		
i. motion			X	
j. anode heel effect	X			
k. patient factors (e.g., size, pathology)	X	X	X	X
l. angle (tube, part, or receptor)			X	X

*'Brightness' when referring to digital images

   B. Technique Charts
   1. caliper measurement
   2. fixed versus variable kVp
   3. special considerations
      a. anatomic and pathologic factors
      b. pediatrics

   C. Image Receptors
   1. system speed
      a. film characteristics
         1. film contrast
         2. film latitude
         3. exposure latitude
      b. screen characteristics
         1. phosphor type
         2. single versus double film/screen system

   2. digital image characteristics
      a. spatial resolution
         1. sampling frequency
         2. pixel size (e.g., detector element size)
         3. receptor size and matrix size
      b. image signal (exposure related)
         1. quantum mottle
         2. SNR (signal to noise ratio)
         3. CNR (contrast to noise ratio)

C. IMAGE PRODUCTION AND EVALUATION (cont.)

II. **Image Processing and Quality Assurance (6)**

A. Film Storage

B. Cassette Loading

C. Image Identification

    1. methods (e.g., photographic, radiographic, electronic)

    2. legal considerations (e.g., patient data, examination data)

D. Automatic Film Processor

    1. components*

        a. developer

        b. fixer

        c. wash

        d. dry

    2. systems

        a. transport

        b. replenishment

        c. temperature regulation

        d. recirculation

        e. dryer

    3. maintenance

        a. start up and shut down procedure

        b. removal and cleaning of crossover assembly

        c. sensitometric monitoring

    4. system malfunction

        a. observable effects (e.g., artifacts, fluctuations in density, contrast)

        b. possible causes (e.g., improper temperature, contamination, roller alignment, replenishment, water flow)

E. Digital Systems

    1. grayscale rendition or look-up table (LUT)

    2. edge enhancement

    3. noise suppression

    4. contrast enhancement

    5. system malfunctions (e.g., ghost image, banding, erasure, dead pixels, readout problems, printer distortion)

F. PACS

    1. DICOM

    2. malfunction (e.g., inappropriate documentation, lost images, mismatched images, corrupt data)

    3. window level and window width

III. **Criteria for Image Evaluation (8)**

A. Density (mAs, distance, film-screen combination)

B. Contrast (kVp, filtration, grids)

C. Recorded Detail (motion, poor film-screen contact)

D. Distortion (magnification, OID, SID)

E. Demonstration of Anatomical Structures (positioning, tube-part-image receptor alignment)

F. Identification Markers (anatomical, patient, date)

G. Patient Considerations (pathologic conditions, motion)

H. Digital and film artifacts (film handling artifacts, static, pressure artifacts, grid lines, Moiré effect or aliasing)

I. Fog (age, chemical, radiation, temperature, safelight)

J. Noise

K. Acceptable Range of Exposure

L. Exposure Indicator Determination

M. Gross Exposure Error

N. Image Degradation (mottle, light or dark, low contrast)

*Specific chemicals in the processing solutions will not be covered (e.g., glutaraldehyde).

D. PATIENT CARE AND EDUCATION (15)

I. Ethical and Legal Aspects (3)

A. Patient's Rights

    1. informed consent (e.g., written, oral, implied)

    2. confidentiality (HIPAA)

    3. additional rights (e.g., Patient's Bill of Rights)
       a. privacy
       b. extent of care (e.g., DNR)
       c. access to information
       d. living will; health care proxy
       e. research participation

B. Legal Issues

    1. examination requisition

    2. common terminology (e.g., battery, negligence, malpractice)

    3. legal doctrines (e.g., *respondeat superior*, *res ipsa loquitur*)

C. Professional Ethics

II. Interpersonal Communication (2)

A. Modes of Communication

    1. verbal/written

    2. nonverbal (e.g., eye contact, touching)

B. Challenges in Communication

    1. patient characteristics

    2. explanation of medical terms

    3. strategies to improve understanding

C. Patient Education (e.g., explanation of current procedure)

III. Infection Control (6)

A. Terminology and Basic Concepts

    1. asepsis
       a. medical
       b. surgical
       c. sterile technique

    2. pathogens
       a. fomites, vehicles, vectors
       b. nosocomial infections

B. Cycle of Infection

    1. pathogen

    2. source or reservoir of infection

    3. susceptible host

    4. method of transmission
       a. contact (direct, indirect)
       b. droplet
       c. airborne/suspended
       d. common vehicle
       e. vector borne

C. Standard Precautions

    1. handwashing

    2. gloves, gowns

    3. masks

    4. medical asepsis (e.g., equipment disinfection)

D. Additional or Transmission-Based Precautions (e.g., hepatitis B, HIV, rubella, tuberculosis)

    1. airborne (e.g., respiratory protection, negative ventilation)

    2. droplet (e.g., particulate mask, restricted patient placement)

    3. contact (e.g., gloves, gown, restricted patient placement)

E. Disposal of Contaminated Materials

    1. linens

    2. needles

    3. patient supplies (e.g., tubes, emesis basin)

IV. Physical Assistance and Transfer (2)

A. Patient Transfer and Movement

    1. body mechanics (balance, alignment, movement)

    2. patient transfer

B. Assisting Patients with Medical Equipment (e.g., oxygen delivery systems)

C. Routine Monitoring

    1. equipment (e.g., stethoscope, sphygmomanometer)

    2. vital signs (e.g., blood pressure, pulse, respiration, temperature)

    3. physical signs and symptoms (e.g., motor control, severity of injury)

    4. documentation

V. Medical Emergencies (2)

A. Allergic Reactions (e.g., latex)

B. Cardiac or Respiratory Arrest (e.g., CPR)

C. Physical Injury or Trauma

D. Other Medical Disorders (e.g., seizures, diabetic reactions)

E. SPECIFIC RADIOGRAPHIC PROCEDURES

The specific positions and projections within each anatomic region that may be covered on the examination are listed in Attachment A. A guide to positioning terminology appears in Attachments B and C.

ANATOMIC MODULE [1]	# QUESTIONS PER MODULE	FOCUS OF QUESTIONS [2]
I. Chest		1. **Positioning** (topographic landmarks, body positions, path of central ray, etc.)
A. Routine	16	emphasis: high
B. Other	4	
TOTAL	20	
II. Extremities		2. **Anatomy** (including physiology, basic pathology, and related medical terminology)
A. Lower (toes, foot, calcaneus, ankle, tibia, fibula, knee, patella, and distal femur)	11	emphasis: medium
B. Upper (fingers, hand, wrist, forearm, elbow, and humerus)	11	
C. Pectoral Girdle (shoulder, scapula, clavicle, and acromioclavicular joints)	3	3. **Technical Factors** [2] (including adjustments for circumstances such as body habitus, trauma, pathology, breathing techniques, casts, splints, etc.)
TOTAL	25	
III. Skull/Sinuses		
A. Skull	8	emphasis: low
B. Paranasal Sinuses	8	
C. Facial Bones (nasal bones, orbits)	4	
TOTAL	20	4. **Equipment and Accessories** (grids or Bucky, compensating filter, automatic exposure control [AEC])
IV. Spine		
A. Cervical Spine	8	emphasis: low
B. Thoracic Spine	6	
C. Lumbosacral Spine	8	
D. Sacrum, Coccyx, and Sacroiliac Joints	2	
E. Scoliosis Series	1	
TOTAL	25	
V. Podiatric [3]		
A. Foot	14	
B. Ankle	5	
C. Calcaneus (Os Calcis)	1	
TOTAL	20	

Notes:

1. Examinees take one or more anatomic modules, depending on the type of license they have applied for. Each anatomic module has 20 or 25 scored test questions, depending on the module (see chart above). The number of questions <u>within</u> a module should be regarded as approximate values.

2. The anatomic modules may include questions about the four areas listed under *FOCUS OF QUESTIONS* on the right side of the chart. The PODIATRIC module does <u>not</u> include questions on any of the *technical factors* or specialized equipment/accessories section.

3. The PODIATRIC module section may include 1 or 2 additional unscored (pilot) questions.

Attachment A
Radiographic Positions and Projections

I. **Chest**
   A. Chest
      1. PA upright
      2. lateral upright
      3. AP lordotic
      4. AP supine
      5. lateral decubitus
      6. posterior oblique
      7. anterior oblique

II. **Extremities**
   A. Toes
      1. AP
      2. oblique
      3. lateral
   B. Foot
      1. AP angle toward heel
      2. medial oblique
      3. lateral oblique
      4. mediolateral
      5. lateromedial
      6. sesamoids, tangential
      7. AP weight bearing
      8. lateral weight bearing
   C. Calcaneus (Os Calcis)
      1. lateral
      2. plantodorsal, axial
      3. dorsoplantar, axial
   D. Ankle
      1. AP
      2. AP mortise
      3. mediolateral
      4. oblique, 45 degrees internal
      5. lateromedial
      6. AP stress views
   E. Tibia, Fibula
      1. AP
      2. lateral
      3. oblique
   F. Knee
      1. AP
      2. lateral
      3. AP weight bearing
      4. lateral oblique 45 degrees
      5. medial oblique 45 degrees
      6. PA
      7. PA axial—intercondylar
         fossa (tunnel)
   G. Patella
      1. lateral
      2. supine flexion 45 degrees
         (Merchant)
      3. PA
      4. prone flexion 90 degrees
         (Settegast)
      5. prone flexion 55 degrees
         (Hughston)
   H. Femur (Distal)
      1. AP
      2. mediolateral
   I. Fingers
      1. PA finger
      2. lateral
      3. oblique
      4. AP thumb
      5. oblique thumb
      6. lateral thumb

   J. Hand
      1. PA
      2. lateral
      3. oblique
   K. Wrist
      1. PA
      2. oblique 45 degrees
      3. lateral
      4. PA for scaphoid
      5. scaphoid (Stecher)
      6. carpal canal
   L. Forearm
      1. AP
      2. lateral
   M. Elbow
      1. AP
      2. lateral
      3. external oblique
      4. internal oblique
      5. AP partial flexion
      6. axial trauma (Coyle)
   N. Humerus
      1. AP
      2. lateral
      3. AP neutral
      4. scapular Y
      5. transthoracic lateral
   O. Shoulder
      1. AP internal and external
         rotation
      2. inferosuperior axial
      3. posterior oblique (Grashey)
      4. tangential
      5. AP neutral
      6. transthoracic lateral
      7. scapular Y
   P. Scapula
      1. AP
      2. lateral, anterior oblique
      3. lateral, posterior oblique
   Q. Clavicle
      1. AP
      2. AP angle 15-30 degrees
         cephalad
      3. PA angle 15-30 degrees
         caudad
   R. Acromioclavicular joints
      1. AP bilateral with and without
         weights

III. **Skull/Sinuses**
   A. Skull
      1. AP axial (Towne)
      2. lateral
      3. PA (Caldwell)
      4. PA
      5. submentovertical
         (full basal)
   B. Facial Bones
      1. lateral
      2. parietoacanthial (Waters)
      3. PA (Caldwell)
      4. PA (modified Waters)
   C. Nasal Bones
      1. parietoacanthial (Waters)
      2. lateral
      3. PA (Caldwell)

   D. Orbits
      1. parietoacanthial (Waters)
      2. lateral
      3. PA (Caldwell)
   E. Paranasal Sinuses
      1. lateral
      2. PA (Caldwell)
      3. parietoacanthial (Waters)
      4. submentovertical (full basal)
      5. open mouth parietoacanthial
         (Waters)

IV. **Spine**
   A. Cervical spine
      1. AP angle cephalad
      2. AP open mouth
      3. lateral
      4. anterior oblique
      5. posterior oblique
      6. lateral swimmers
      7. lateral flexion and extension
   B. Thoracic Spine
      1. AP
      2. lateral, breathing
      3. lateral, expiration
   C. Lumbar Spine
      1. AP
      2. PA
      3. lateral
      4. L5-S1 lateral spot
      5. posterior oblique 45 degrees
      6. anterior oblique 45 degrees
      7. AP L5-S1, 30-35 degrees
         cephalad
      8. AP right and left bending
      9. lateral flexion and extension
   C. Sacrum and Coccyx
      1. AP sacrum, 15-25 degrees
         cephalad
      2. AP coccyx, 10-20 degrees caudad
      3. lateral sacrum and coccyx,
         combined
      4. lateral sacrum or coccyx,
         separate
   D. Sacroiliac Joints
      1. AP
      2. posterior oblique
      3. anterior oblique
   E. Scoliosis Series
      1. AP/PA scoliosis series
         (Ferguson)

V. **Podiatric**
   A. Foot
      1. dorsal plantar (DP)
      2. medial oblique
      3. lateral oblique
      4. lateral
      5. sesamoidal axial
   B. Ankle
      1. AP
      2. AP mortise
      3. AP medial oblique
      4. AP lateral oblique
      5. lateral
   C. Calcaneus (Os Calcis)
      1. axial calcaneal
      2. Harris and Beath (ski-jump)

Attachment B
Standard Terminology
for Positioning and Projection

Radiographic View: Describes the body part as seen by the x-ray film or other recording medium, such as a fluoroscopic screen. Restricted to the discussion of a <u>radiograph</u> or <u>image</u>.

Radiographic Position: Refers to a specific body position, such as supine, prone, recumbent, erect, or Trendelenburg. Restricted to the discussion of the <u>patient's physical position</u>.

Radiographic Projection: Restricted to the discussion of the <u>path of the central ray</u>.

POSITIONING TERMINOLOGY

A. Lying Down

1. *supine*   –   lying on the back
2. *prone*   –   lying face downward
3. *decubitus*   –   lying down with a horizontal x-ray beam
4. *recumbent*   –   lying down in any position

B. Erect or Upright

1. *anterior position*   –   facing the film
2. *posterior position* –   facing the radiographic tube
3. *oblique position*   –   (erect or lying down)

   a. anterior (facing the film)

   i. *left anterior oblique*   body rotated with the left anterior portion closest to the film.
   ii. *right anterior oblique*   body rotated with the right anterior portion closest to the film

   b. posterior (facing the radiographic tube)

   i. *left posterior oblique*   body rotated with the left posterior portion closest to the film.
   ii. *right posterior oblique*   body rotated with the right posterior portion closest to the film

Attachment C

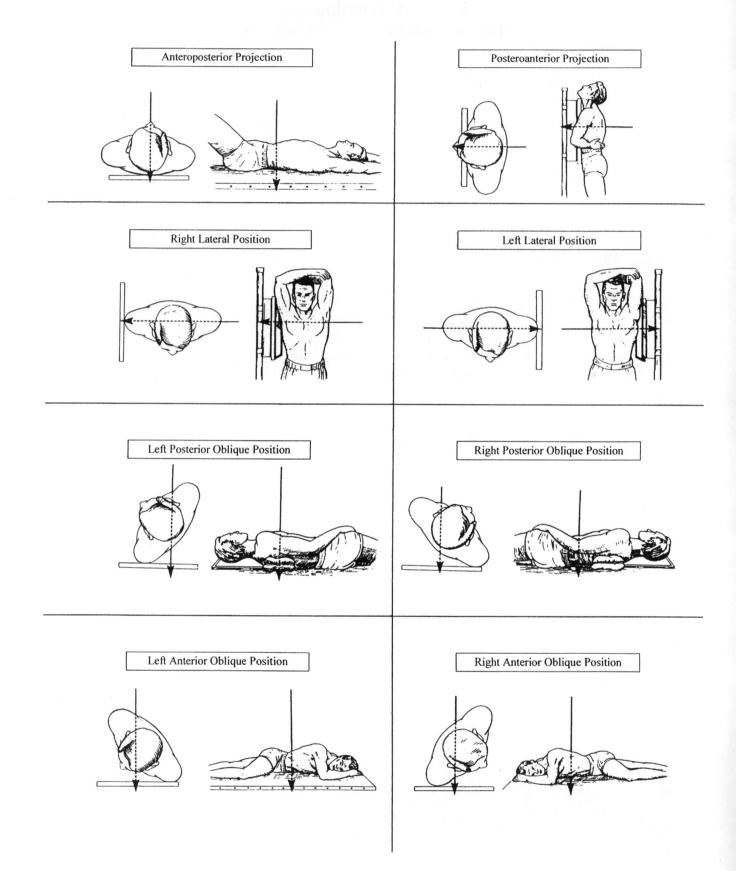

Attachment D
ARRT Standard Definitions

Term	Film-Screen Radiography	Term	Digital Radiography
Recorded Detail	The sharpness of the structural lines as recorded in the radiographic image.	Recorded Detail	The sharpness of the structural edges recorded in the image.
Density	Radiographic density is the degree of blackening or opacity of an area in a radiograph due to the accumulation of black metallic silver following exposure and processing of a film. $\text{Density} = \text{Log} \dfrac{\text{incident light intensity}}{\text{transmitted light intensity}}$	Brightness	Brightness is the measurement of the luminance of a monitor calibrated in units of candela (cd) per square meter on a monitor or soft copy. Density on a hard copy is the same as film.
Contrast	Radiographic contrast is defined as the visible differences between any two selected areas of density levels within the radiographic image. *Scale of Contrast* refers to the number of densities visible (or the number of shades of gray). *Long Scale* is the term used when slight differences between densities are present (low contrast) but the total number of densities is increased. *Short Scale* is the term used when considerable or major differences between densities are present (high contrast) but the total number of densities is reduced.	Contrast	Image contrast or display contrast is determined primarily by the processing algorithm (mathematical codes used by the software to provide the desired image appearance). The default algorithm determines the initial processing codes applied to the image data. *Scale of Contrast* is synonymous to "gray scale" and is linked to the bit depth of the system. 'Gray scale' is used instead of 'scale of contrast' when referring to digital images.
Film Latitude	The inherent ability of the film to record a long range of density levels on the radiograph. Film latitude and film contrast depend upon the sensitometric properties of the film and the processing conditions and are determined directly from the characteristic H and D curve.	Dynamic Range	The range of exposures that may be captured by a detector. The dynamic range for digital imaging is much larger than film.
Film Contrast	The inherent ability of the film emulsion to react to radiation and record a range of densities.	Receptor Contrast	The fixed characteristic of the receptor. Most digital receptors have an essentially linear response to exposure. This is impacted by **contrast resolution** (the smallest exposure change or signal difference that can be detected). Ultimately, contrast resolution is limited by the dynamic range and the **quantization** (number of bits per pixel) of the detector.
Exposure Latitude	The range of exposure factors which will produce a diagnostic radiograph.	Exposure Latitude	The range of exposures which produces quality images at appropriate patient dose.
Subject Contrast	The difference in the quantity of radiation transmitted by a particular part as a result of the different absorption characteristics of the tissues and structures making up that part.	Subject Contrast	The magnitude of the signal difference in the remnant beam.

Simulated Examination for the Limited Scope of Practice in Radiography

Simulated Examination for the Limited Scope of Practice in Radiography—Core Module

Complete this examination in pencil, if you plan to take it more than once. If you are not sure of the answer to a question, skip it and return to it after completing the entire examination.

Multiple Choice

Identify the choice that best completes the statement or answers the question.

_____ 1. Which of the following statements are correct regarding the link between radiation dose and genetic effects?
    1. The link has been demonstrated in human studies.
    2. The link has been demonstrated in animal studies.
    3. Increased risk to humans cannot be predicted with respect to an individual.
    A. 1 and 2 only
    B. 1 and 3 only
    C. 2 and 3 only
    D. 1, 2, and 3

_____ 2. Which of the following changes in kilovoltage (kVp) will result in the greatest reduction of patient dose, when milliampere-seconds (mAs) is adjusted to compensate for the change?
    A. Decrease kVp by 30%
    B. Decrease kVp by 15%
    C. Increase kVp by 15%
    D. Increase kVp by 30%

_____ 3. Which of the following image receptor (IR) system speeds will result in the lowest patient dose?
    A. Slower-speed IR system
    B. Faster-speed IR system
    C. Doesn't matter—IR system speed doesn't effect patient dose

_____ 4. What is the primary purpose of using gonad shields during radiography?
    A. Reduce the likelihood of genetic effects
    B. Reduce the likelihood of somatic effects
    C. Protect patient modesty
    D. Demonstrate the location of the gonads in the image

_____ 5. Which of the following are types of gonad shields?
    1. Aperture
    2. Contact
    3. Shadow
    A. 1 and 2 only
    B. 1 and 3 only
    C. 2 and 3 only
    D. 1, 2, and 3

_____ 6. When should gonad shielding be used?
    A. For all patients
    B. For all procedures
    C. When the gonads are within 10 cm of the radiation field
    D. When the gonads are within 5 cm of the radiation field

____ 7. The greatest cause of unnecessary radiation to patients that can be controlled by the limited operator is:
A. patient condition.
B. patient size.
C. repeat exposures.
D. equipment malfunction.

____ 8. The limited operator can reduce repeat exposures by:
A. accepting marginal images.
B. clearly instructing patients.
C. increasing source-image distance (SID).
D. optimizing kVp.

____ 9. How does x-ray beam restriction minimize patient exposure?
A. Limits radiation fog
B. Limits the radiation field to the area of interest
C. Limits effect of patient motion
D. Limits repeat exposures

____ 10. What is the device that allows the limited operator to vary the size of the radiation field?
A. Collimator
B. Detent
C. Filter
D. Shield

____ 11. How does filtration reduce patient exposure?
A. Removes shorter-wavelength photons
B. Removes longer-wavelength photons
C. Reduces the size of the radiation field
D. Reduces the time of exposure

____ 12. What is the National Council on Radiation Protection and Measurements (NCRP) recommendation for the amount of total filtration?
A. 0.5 mm aluminum equivalent (Al equiv)
B. 1.5 mm Al equiv
C. 2.5 mm Al equiv
D. 3.5 mm Al equiv

____ 13. What are the three principal methods used to protect limited operators from unnecessary radiation exposure?
A. Time, distance, shielding
B. Time, distance, collimation
C. Distance, collimation, shielding
D. Time, collimation, filtration

____ 14. Which of the following is *not* a type of personnel radiation shielding?
A. Apron
B. Glove
C. Thyroid shield
D. Shadow

____ 15. Personnel shielding must be worn on the rare occasion on which the limited operator may need to remain in the radiographic room during an exposure to assist the patient in maintaining the proper position. What is the source of the greatest radiation hazard under this circumstance?
A. Off-focus radiation
B. Leakage radiation
C. Scattered radiation from the patient
D. Backscatter radiation from the IR

____ 16. What is the term for radiation that escapes from the x-ray tube housing?
A. Scattered radiation
B. Off-focus radiation
C. Primary radiation
D. Leakage

____ 17. Why are limited operators prohibited from activities that result in direct exposure to the primary x-ray beam?
A. They are considered occupationally exposed individuals.
B. These activities carry immediate health risks.
C. Their interaction with the beam will affect patient dose.
D. Their presence near the patient increases liability.

____ 18. Distance, as a method used to limit operator exposure, means that:
A. the operator should maximize the distance from the source during an exposure.
B. the operator should minimize the distance from the source during an exposure.
C. the operator should maximize the distance from the patient during an exposure.
D. the operator should minimize the distance from the patient during an exposure.

____ 19. Shielding worn for personnel protection is designed to attenuate what source of exposure?
A. Primary
B. Off focus
C. Leakage
D. Scatter

_____ 20. Which of the following is an acronym for a common type of personnel dosimeter?
A. TLC
B. TLD
C. OSD
D. OID

_____ 21. What is the recommended placement for a personnel dosimeter on the body of the limited operator?
A. Badge should be worn in the region of the waist on the anterior surface of the body and outside the lead apron, if worn.
B. Badge should be worn in the region of the waist on the posterior surface of the body and inside the lead apron, if worn.
C. Badge should be worn in the region of the collar on the posterior surface of the body and inside the lead apron, if worn.
D. Badge should be worn in the region of the collar on the anterior surface of the body and outside the lead apron, if worn.

_____ 22. What is the NCRP recommended annual effective dose limit for occupational exposure?
A. 0.05 rem
B. 0.5 rem
C. 5.0 rem
D. 50.0 rem

_____ 23. What is the NCRP recommended monthly effective (or equivalent) dose limit to the fetus for a pregnant worker?
A. 0.05 rem
B. 0.5 rem
C. 5.0 rem
D. 50.0 rem

_____ 24. Radiation monitoring of personnel is required when what percentage of the annual occupational effective dose limit is likely to be received?
A. 5%
B. 10%
C. 15%
D. 20%

_____ 25. What is the conventional (British system) radiation unit to express radiation intensity in air?
A. Coulomb/kilogram (C/kg)
B. Watt
C. Ohm
D. Roentgen

_____ 26. The conventional (British system) unit commonly used to report occupational dose to radiation workers in the United States is the:
A. mR.
B. rad.
C. rem.
D. mGy.

_____ 27. What is the conventional (British system) radiation unit of absorbed dose?
A. Rad
B. Roentgen
C. Gray
D. Rem

_____ 28. According to the Bergonié-Tribondeau law, which of the following types of cells are most radiosensitive?
A. Brain cells
B. Embryonic tissue
C. Cells of the gastric mucosa
D. Skin cells

_____ 29. Which of the following types of radiation effects is typical of the risk to a patient undergoing a diagnostic x-ray examination?
A. Short-term effects
B. Genetic effects
C. Nonstochastic effects
D. Stochastic effects

_____ 30. Which of the following occur with high radiation doses?
1. Stochastic effects
2. Short-term somatic effects
3. Nonstochastic effects
A. 1 and 2 only
B. 1 and 3 only
C. 2 and 3 only
D. 1, 2, and 3

_____ 31. What is erythema?
A. Loss of hair caused by a high radiation dose
B. Loss of hair caused by long-term low radiation dose
C. Reddening of the skin caused by high radiation dose
D. Reddening of the skin caused by long-term low radiation dose

_____ 32. What is the guiding philosophy of radiation protection?
A. ALARMA—as long as radiographs are made accessible
B. ALARA—as low as reasonably achievable
C. ALAIS—as long as ionizations are small
D. ALAP—as low as possible

____ 33. Which of the following statements reflects current scientific opinion regarding the effects of diagnostic levels of ionizing radiation?
A. It is carcinogenic after a certain number of examinations have been performed.
B. Spontaneous abortion will occur if the patient is pregnant.
C. Depression of the white blood cell count is followed by acute gastrointestinal distress.
D. There is increased risk of cancer, leukemia, birth defects, and cataracts.

____ 34. Which of the following changes will decrease patient dose?
1. Using faster intensifying screens
2. Increasing the kVp using the 15% rule
3. Increasing the grid ratio to a 16:1 ratio
A. 1 and 2 only
B. 1 and 3 only
C. 2 and 3 only
D. 1, 2, and 3

____ 35. When radiation exposure occurs during pregnancy, the greatest risk of birth defects occurs when the exposure:
1. exceeds 5 rad to the uterus.
2. occurs within the first trimester of pregnancy.
3. occurs within the third trimester of pregnancy.
A. 1 and 2 only
B. 1 and 3 only
C. 2 and 3 only
D. 1, 2, and 3

____ 36. What are the four essential elements required for x-ray production?
A. A target, a vacuum, an electron source, and a high potential difference
B. A target, an electron source, an inert gas environment, and a high potential difference
C. An electron source, a magnetic field, a resistance-free path, and a target
D. An electron source, an electric field, a circuit, and a target

____ 37. The target of the x-ray tube is made of:
A. tungsten.
B. glass.
C. stainless steel.
D. fluorescent phosphors.

____ 38. The greatest portion of the x-ray beam is made up of:
A. characteristic radiation.
B. bremsstrahlung radiation.
C. electrons.
D. heat.

____ 39. The penetrating power of the x-ray beam is controlled by varying the:
A. anode angle.
B. anode speed.
C. milliamperage (mA).
D. kilovoltage (kVp).

____ 40. Which of the following functions involve the autotransformer?
A. kVp selection
B. mA selection
C. Exposure time selection
D. Automatic exposure control

____ 41. The process of causing alternating current to flow in one direction only is called:
A. rectification.
B. induction.
C. grounding.
D. compensation.

____ 42. Nearly all new x-ray machines manufactured today use _____ generators.
A. single-phase
B. three-phase, 6-pulse
C. three-phase, 12-pulse
D. high-frequency

____ 43. What is the standard control limit for the field light to radiation field alignment test?
A. Exact alignment
B. ±1% of SID
C. ±2% of SID
D. ±5% of SID

____ 44. What is the standard control limit for the beam (central ray) alignment test?
A. Exact alignment
B. Within 1 degree of perpendicular
C. Within 2 degree of perpendicular
D. Within 5 degree of perpendicular

____ 45. How often should lead aprons and gloves be checked for cracks or holes?
A. Every 3 months
B. Every 6 months
C. Every 9 months
D. Every 12 months

_____ 46. At what kVp levels do Compton interactions occur?
A. They don't occur with x-ray exposure
B. Below the diagnostic radiology kVp range
C. Above the diagnostic radiology kVp range
D. Throughout the diagnostic radiology kVp range

_____ 47. Which of the following is used to test film/screen contact?
A. Wire mesh tool
B. Densitometer
C. Sensitometer
D. H & D curve

_____ 48. Which of the following are the prime factors of exposure in radiography?
A. Density, contrast, recorded detail, and distortion
B. Density, contrast, distortion, and kVp
C. mAs, kVp, density, and distance (SID)
D. mA, exposure time, kVp, and distance (SID)

_____ 49. Which of the following will result in increased radiographic density?
1. Increased mA
2. Increased exposure time
3. Increased kVp
A. 1 and 2 only
B. 1 and 3 only
C. 2 and 3 only
D. 1, 2, and 3

_____ 50. If the radiographic image is overexposed, which of the following changes in exposure factors should be used to correct the problem?
A. Decrease kVp
B. Increase kVp
C. Increase mAs
D. Decrease mAs

_____ 51. The relationship between SID and beam intensity is expressed in the:
A. proportional square law.
B. inverse square law.
C. reciprocity law.
D. target-distance law.

_____ 52. What are the four primary aspects of radiographic quality?
A. mA, seconds, kVp, and SID
B. SID, density, contrast, and mAs
C. Density, contrast, distortion, and recorded detail
D. Density, contrast, distortion, and distance

_____ 53. Contrast is primarily controlled by altering the:
A. mA.
B. exposure time.
C. kVp.
D. mAs.

_____ 54. Fog affects radiographic quality by causing:
A. underexposure.
B. decreased contrast.
C. increased contrast.
D. decreased density.

_____ 55. A change from the small focal spot to the large focal spot will result in:
A. decreased image sharpness.
B. magnification.
C. distortion.
D. increased contrast.

_____ 56. An increase in object-image distance (OID) will result in:
A. increased magnification.
B. increased image sharpness.
C. loss of contrast.
D. increased radiographic density.

_____ 57. Motion of the patient, the tube, or the IR during the exposure will result in decreased:
A. contrast.
B. distortion.
C. radiographic density.
D. recorded detail.

_____ 58. Quantum mottle or graininess in the radiographic image because of the size and distribution of film and/or screen crystals affects image quality by decreasing the radiographic:
A. density.
B. recorded detail.
C. contrast.
D. latitude.

_____ 59. Quantum mottle is only a problem with:
A. low kVp exposures.
B. poor film/screen contact.
C. very slow speed IR systems.
D. very fast speed IR systems.

_____ 60. Which of the following will increase recorded detail?
1. Increase in SID
2. Increase in OID
3. Decrease in focal spot size
A. 1 and 2 only
B. 1 and 3 only
C. 2 and 3 only
D. 1, 2, and 3

_____ 61. Intensifying screen speed is defined as:
A. the color of light emitted by a screen.
B. the ability to emit light when exposed to x-rays.
C. the optical density minus the base + fog value.
D. the efficiency of a screen in converting x-rays to light.

_____ 62. What is the proper method for storing unopened boxes of x-ray film?
A. Stacked flat with edges of boxes aligned
B. Stacked flat with edges of boxes staggered
C. Standing on edge
D. X-ray film cannot be safely stored

_____ 63. Which of the following describe the characteristic curve of a film with wide latitude and longer scale contrast?
A. A steep, vertical curve
B. A more horizontal and wide curve
C. A curve that plots closer to the left of the graph
D. A curve that plots closer to the right of the graph

_____ 64. What controls the amount of replenisher added in automatic processing?
A. Timers on the replenishment pumps
B. The limited operator
C. The size of the film passing over an intake sensor
D. The strength of the developer as measured by the sensitometer

_____ 65. Which of the following is the correct sequence of the steps in automatic processing?
A. Developer, wash, fixer, wash, dry
B. Developer, fixer, wash, dry
C. Developer, wash, fixer, dry
D. Wash, developer, fixer, dry

_____ 66. What two specialized instruments are required for monitoring processor performance?
A. Densitometer and sensitometer
B. Densitometer and dosimeter
C. Sensitometer and dosimeter
D. Dosimeter and thermometer

_____ 67. Marks, exposures, or images on a radiograph that are not a part of the intended image are called:
A. fog.
B. ghosts.
C. phantoms.
D. artifacts.

_____ 68. Which of the following factors affect the quantity of scatter radiation fog on a radiograph?
1. Field size
2. Focal spot size
3. kVp
A. 1 and 2 only
B. 1 and 3 only
C. 2 and 3 only
D. 1, 2, and 3

_____ 69. If the size of the x-ray field increases, what happens to scatter radiation fog?
A. Scatter radiation fog increases also.
B. Scatter radiation fog decreases.
C. Scatter radiation fog is not affected by field size.
D. The effect of field size on scatter radiation fog is dependent on the focal spot size used in making the exposure.

_____ 70. If the amount of irradiated tissue increases, what happens to scatter radiation fog?
A. There is not enough information provided to answer the question.
B. Scatter radiation fog increases.
C. Scatter radiation fog decreases.
D. Scatter radiation fog is not affected by the amount of tissue irradiated.

_____ 71. What is the principal source of scatter radiation in radiography?
A. The tube housing
B. The patient
C. The IR
D. The collimator

_____ 72. The most effective and practical way to reduce scatter radiation fog on a radiograph is to:
A. decrease the OID.
B. decrease the SID.
C. increase the kVp.
D. use a grid or Bucky.

_____ 73. As a general rule, a grid should be employed when the part thickness is greater than:
A. 4 cm.
B. 12 cm.
C. 18 cm.
D. 12 inches.

_____ 74. Technique charts are based on patient part measurements obtained using an x-ray caliper and are expressed as:
A. circumference in inches.
B. thickness in centimeters.
C. diameter in millimeters.
D. depth in inches.

_____ 75. Which of the following pathologic conditions would require a decrease in exposure?
1. Multiple myeloma
2. Emphysema
3. Osteoporosis
A. 1 and 2 only
B. 1 and 3 only
C. 2 and 3 only
D. 1, 2, and 3

_____ 76. How will the anode heel effect, if present, be seen on an image?
A. Image will have higher contrast on the anode end than on the cathode end.
B. Image will have lower contrast on the anode end than on the cathode end.
C. Image will be darker on the anode end than on the cathode end.
D. Image will be lighter on the anode end than on the cathode end.

_____ 77. Which radiographic quality factor is most affected by angulation of the central ray, part, or IR?
A. Density
B. Contrast
C. Detail
D. Distortion

_____ 78. What is the recommendation for a hard-copy image that is mislabeled?
A. The image must be repeated to ensure a correct, permanent label.
B. A sticker with the correct information should be applied to the hard-copy image.
C. The correct information should be hand written on the hard-copy image.
D. No correction is needed.

_____ 79. Which of the following will result in a screen/film image with insufficient density?
A. Use of a relative speed (RS) 100 screen with the mAs set for an RS 300 screen
B. Use of an RS 300 screen with the mAs set for an RS 100 screen
C. IR exposure at an SID closer than expected for the exposure factors selected
D. IR exposure with an mAs less than needed for the particular anatomic structures

_____ 80. Which of the following will result in a screen/film image with insufficient contrast?
A. Use of an RS 100 screen with the mAs set for an RS 300 screen
B. Use of an RS 300 screen with the mAs set for an RS 100 screen
C. IR exposure at an SID closer than expected for the exposure factors selected
D. IR exposure with a kVp higher than needed for the particular anatomic structures

_____ 81. Which of the following will result in a screen/film image with poor recorded detail?
A. Use of an RS 100 screen with the mAs set for an RS 300 screen
B. Use of an RS 300 screen with the mAs set for an RS 100 screen
C. Poor screen and film contact in the IR
D. IR exposure with the mAs higher than needed for the particular anatomic structures

_____ 82. Which of the following will result in a screen/film image with poor recorded detail?
A. Use of an RS 100 screen with the mAs set for an RS 300 screen
B. IR exposure with an mAs higher than needed for the particular anatomic structures
C. IR exposure with a kVp higher than needed for the particular anatomic structures
D. Patient motion

_____ 83. Which of the following will result in a screen/film image with excessive magnification of image structures?
A. Use of an RS 100 screen with the mAs set for an RS 300 screen
B. IR exposure at an SID greater than recommended for a particular body part
C. IR exposure at an OID greater than recommended for a particular body part
D. IR exposure with an mAs higher than needed for the particular anatomic structures

_____ 84. Which of the following will result in a screen/film image with excessive distortion of image structures?
A. Improper positioning of the anatomic structure on the IR
B. Use of an 8:1 grid with the mAs set for a 12:1 grid
C. IR exposure at an SID greater than recommended for a particular body part
D. IR exposure with the mAs higher than needed for the particular anatomic structures

_____ 85. Which screen/film image artifact looks like lightning?
A. Static artifact
B. Handling artifact
C. Pressure artifact
D. Chemical artifact

_____ 86. Which of the following would be a violation of patient confidentiality?
A. A limited operator discusses a patient's existing pathology with a radiographer to get assistance in setting technical factors.
B. A limited operator talks to his friend during lunch about a patient's imaging procedure.
C. A radiographer asks if a patient is pregnant before an acute abdominal series.
D. A transporter tells the limited operator that the patient complained of dizziness while riding in the wheelchair to the x-ray department.

_____ 87. Which of the following are true regarding informed consent?
1. Informed consent may be revoked at any time.
2. The patient must be legally competent to sign.
3. The patient may sign an incomplete form and the blanks may be filled in later by the physician.
A. 1 and 2 only
B. 1 and 3 only
C. 2 and 3 only
D. 1, 2, and 3 only

_____ 88. A limited operator innocently commits an error as a result of following the orders of his or her employer, a physician. The employer may be held responsible according to the:
A. American Society of Radiologic Technologists code of ethics.
B. rule of professional responsibility.
C. doctrine of *respondeat superior*.
D. doctrine of *non compos mentis*.

_____ 89. Communication has been "validated" when the speaker has:
A. spoken clearly.
B. received a response from the listener that demonstrates comprehension.
C. presented the information accurately.
D. reviewed the material.

_____ 90. Mrs. Elizabeth Dunbar is 86 years old and a bit confused. She is most likely to respond appropriately if you address her as:
A. Betty.
B. Honey.
C. Mrs. Dunbar.
D. Elizabeth.

_____ 91. Which of the following are correct statements of proper body mechanics?
1. Use a broad stance.
2. Turn and lift using your back muscles.
3. Carry heavy objects close to your body.
A. 1 and 2 only
B. 1 and 3 only
C. 2 and 3 only
D. 1, 2, and 3

_____ 92. Which term refers to any medium that transports microorganisms?
A. Vehicle
B. Vector
C. Fomite
D. Cycle of infection

_____ 93. What type of disease transmission is possible when the limited operator does not clean the Bucky device after performing an examination on a patient with influenza?
A. Vector transmission
B. Direct contact transmission
C. Fomite transmission
D. Airborne transmission

_____ 94. Standard precautions involve the use of barriers whenever contact is anticipated with:
1. blood.
2. body fluids.
3. mucous membranes.
A. 1 and 2 only
B. 1 and 3 only
C. 2 and 3 only
D. 1, 2, and 3

_____ 95. The process of reducing the probability that infectious organisms will be transmitted to a susceptible individual is called:
A. sepsis.
B. asepsis.
C. disinfection.
D. vaccination.

____ 96. A health care worker's single best protection against disease is:
A. frequent hand hygiene.
B. vaccination.
C. barrier techniques.
D. protective masks.

____ 97. A limited operator who does not change linens between patients is:
A. providing an opportunity for fomite transmission.
B. saving money in laundry expenses.
C. making wise decisions, as long as there are no stains on the linens.
D. increasing productivity by saving time between patients.

____ 98. What is anaphylaxis?
A. The absence of a pain response
B. A severe allergic reaction
C. Complete unconsciousness
D. Inability to breathe

____ 99. Which of the following are symptoms of shock?
1. Cool, clammy skin
2. Increased pulse rate
3. Confusion
A. 1 and 2only
B. 1 and 3 only
C. 2 and 3 only
D. 1, 2, and 3

____ 100. What is the most common site for palpation of a patient's pulse?
A. Carotid artery
B. Apex of the heart
C. Dorsalis pedis
D. Radial artery at the wrist

Simulated Examination for the Limited Scope of Practice in Radiography—Core Module

Answer Section

Multiple Choice

1. **ANS: C**	REF: Ch. 13	OBJ: exam spec A.I.E.1	TOP: radiation biology
2. **ANS: D**	REF: Ch. 13	OBJ: exam spec A.II.A.1	TOP: patient exposure
3. **ANS: B**	REF: Ch. 13	OBJ: exam spec A.II.F	TOP: patient exposure
4. **ANS: A**	REF: Ch. 13	OBJ: exam spec A.II.B.1	TOP: patient exposure
5. **ANS: C**	REF: Ch. 13	OBJ: exam spec A.II.B.2	TOP: patient exposure
6. **ANS: D**	REF: Ch. 13	OBJ: exam spec A.II.B.3	TOP: patient exposure
7. **ANS: C**	REF: Ch. 13	OBJ: exam spec A.II.E	TOP: patient exposure
8. **ANS: B**	REF: Ch. 13	OBJ: exam spec A.II.E.2	TOP: patient exposure
9. **ANS: B**	REF: Ch. 13	OBJ: exam spec A.II.C.1	TOP: patient exposure
10. **ANS: A**	REF: Ch. 2	OBJ: exam spec A.II.C.2	TOP: patient exposure
11. **ANS: B**	REF: Ch. 5	OBJ: exam spec A.II.D.2	TOP: patient exposure
12. **ANS: C**	REF: Ch. 5	OBJ: exam spec A.II.D.3	TOP: patient exposure
13. **ANS: A**	REF: Ch. 13	OBJ: exam spec A.III.B	TOP: personnel protection
14. **ANS: D**	REF: Ch. 13	OBJ: exam spec A.III.C.1	TOP: personnel protection
15. **ANS: C**	REF: Ch. 13	OBJ: exam spec A.III.A.3	TOP: personnel protection
16. **ANS: D**	REF: Ch. 13	OBJ: exam spec A.III.A.2.b	TOP: personnel protection
17. **ANS: A**	REF: Ch. 13	OBJ: exam spec A.III.A.1	TOP: personnel protection
18. **ANS: A**	REF: Ch. 13	OBJ: exam spec A.III.B.2	TOP: personnel protection
19. **ANS: D**	REF: Ch. 13	OBJ: exam spec A.III.A.2.a	TOP: personnel protection
20. **ANS: B**	REF: Ch. 13	OBJ: exam spec A.IV.B.1	TOP: radiation monitoring
21. **ANS: D**	REF: Ch. 13	OBJ: exam spec A.IV.B.2	TOP: radiation monitoring
22. **ANS: C**	REF: Ch. 13	OBJ: exam spec A.IV.C.1	TOP: radiation exposure
23. **ANS: A**	REF: Ch. 13	OBJ: exam spec A.IV.C.3	TOP: radiation exposure
24. **ANS: B**	REF: Ch. 13	OBJ: exam spec A.IV.C.4	TOP: radiation monitoring
25. **ANS: D**	REF: Ch. 13	OBJ: exam spec A.IV.A.3	TOP: radiation exposure
26. **ANS: C**	REF: Ch. 13	OBJ: exam spec A.VI.A.2	TOP: radiation exposure
27. **ANS: A**	REF: Ch. 13	OBJ: exam spec A.VI.A.1	TOP: radiation exposure

28. **ANS: B**	REF: Ch. 13	OBJ: exam spec A.I.A.2	TOP: radiation biology
29. **ANS: D**	REF: Ch. 13	OBJ: exam spec A.I.B	TOP: radiation biology
30. **ANS: C**	REF: Ch. 13	OBJ: exam spec A.I.B	TOP: radiation biology
31. **ANS: C**	REF: Ch. 13	OBJ: exam spec A.I.C.3	TOP: radiation biology
32. **ANS: B**	REF: Ch. 13	OBJ: exam spec A.III.B	TOP: personnel protection
33. **ANS: D**	REF: Ch. 13	OBJ: exam spec A.I.E	TOP: radiation biology
34. **ANS: A**	REF: Ch. 13	OBJ: exam spec A.II.A/F	TOP: patient exposure
35. **ANS: A**	REF: Ch. 13	OBJ: exam spec A.I.D	TOP: radiation biology
36. **ANS: A**	REF: Ch. 5	OBJ: exam spec B.I.A	TOP: radiation physics
37. **ANS: A**	REF: Ch. 5	OBJ: exam spec B.II.A.2.b	TOP: radiographic equipment
38. **ANS: B**	REF: Ch. 5	OBJ: exam spec B.I.B.1	TOP: radiation physics
39. **ANS: D**	REF: Ch. 5	OBJ: exam spec B.I.C.2.a	TOP: radiation physics
40. **ANS: A**	REF: Ch. 6	OBJ: exam spec B.II.B.1	TOP: radiographic equipment
41. **ANS: A**	REF: Ch. 6	OBJ: exam spec B.II.B.1	TOP: radiographic equipment
42. **ANS: D**	REF: Ch. 6	OBJ: exam spec B.II.B.2	TOP: radiographic equipment
43. **ANS: C**	REF: Ch. 11	OBJ: exam spec B.III.A.1	TOP: equipment quality control
44. **ANS: B**	REF: Ch. 11	OBJ: exam spec B.III.A.2	TOP: equipment quality control
45. **ANS: B**	REF: Ch. 13	OBJ: exam spec B.III.D	TOP: accessories quality control
46. **ANS: D**	REF: Ch. 11	OBJ: exam spec B.I.D.1	TOP: radiation physics
47. **ANS: A**	REF: Ch. 8	OBJ: exam spec B.III.C.2	TOP: equipment quality control
48. **ANS: D**	REF: Ch. 7	OBJ: exam spec C.I.A	TOP: technical factor selection
49. **ANS: D**	REF: Ch. 7	OBJ: exam spec C.I.A.b	TOP: technical factor selection
50. **ANS: D**	REF: Ch. 7	OBJ: exam spec C.I.A.a	TOP: technical factor selection
51. **ANS: B**	REF: Ch. 7	OBJ: exam spec C.I.A.d	TOP: technical factor selection
52. **ANS: C**	REF: Ch. 7	OBJ: exam spec C.I.A	TOP: technical factor selection
53. **ANS: C**	REF: Ch. 7	OBJ: exam spec C.I.A.b	TOP: technical factor selection
54. **ANS: B**	REF: Ch. 7	OBJ: exam spec C.III.i	TOP: image evaluation
55. **ANS: A**	REF: Ch. 7	OBJ: exam spec C.I.A.e	TOP: technical factor selection
56. **ANS: A**	REF: Ch. 7	OBJ: exam spec C.I.A.c	TOP: technical factor selection
57. **ANS: D**	REF: Ch. 7	OBJ: exam spec C.I.A.i	TOP: technical factor selection
58. **ANS: B**	REF: Ch. 7	OBJ: exam spec C.I.A.g	TOP: technical factor selection
59. **ANS: D**	REF: Ch. 7	OBJ: exam spec C.I.A.g	TOP: technical factor selection
60. **ANS: B**	REF: Ch. 7	OBJ: exam spec C.I.A.d	TOP: technical factor selection
61. **ANS: D**	REF: Ch. 8	OBJ: exam spec C.I.C.b.2	TOP: technical factor selection
62. **ANS: C**	REF: Ch. 8	OBJ: exam spec C.II.A	TOP: proccessing quality assurance
63. **ANS: B**	REF: Ch. 8	OBJ: exam spec C.I.C.1.a	TOP: image receptors
64. **ANS: C**	REF: Ch. 10	OBJ: exam spec C.II.D.2.b	TOP: film processing
65. **ANS: B**	REF: Ch. 10	OBJ: exam spec C.II.D.1	TOP: film processing
66. **ANS: A**	REF: Ch. 10	OBJ: exam spec C.II.D.3.c	TOP: film processing
67. **ANS: D**	REF: Ch. 10	OBJ: exam spec C.II.D.4.a	TOP: film processing
68. **ANS: B**	REF: Ch. 11	OBJ: exam spec C.I.A.h	TOP: technical factor selection
69. **ANS: A**	REF: Ch. 11	OBJ: exam spec C.I.A.h	TOP: technical factor selection
70. **ANS: B**	REF: Ch. 11	OBJ: exam spec C.I.A.k	TOP: technical factor selection
71. **ANS: B**	REF: Ch. 11	OBJ: exam spec C.I.A.k	TOP: technical factor selection
72. **ANS: D**	REF: Ch. 11	OBJ: exam spec C.I.A.f	TOP: technical factor selection
73. **ANS: B**	REF: Ch. 11	OBJ: exam spec C.I.A.f	TOP: technical factor selection
74. **ANS: B**	REF: Ch. 12	OBJ: exam spec C.I.B.1	TOP: technique charts
75. **ANS: D**	REF: Ch. 12	OBJ: exam spec C.I.B.3.a	TOP: technique charts
76. **ANS: D**	REF: Ch. 5	OBJ: exam spec C.I.A.j	TOP: radiographic quality factors
77. **ANS: D**	REF: Ch. 7	OBJ: exam spec C.I.A.l	TOP: radiographic quality factors
78. **ANS: B**	REF: Ch. 21	OBJ: exam spec C.II.C.2	TOP: image QA
79. **ANS: A**	REF: Ch. 13	OBJ: exam spec C.III.A	TOP: image evaluation
80. **ANS: D**	REF: Ch. 13	OBJ: exam spec C.III.B	TOP: image evaluation
81. **ANS: C**	REF: Ch. 8	OBJ: exam spec C.III.C	TOP: image evaluation
82. **ANS: D**	REF: Ch. 21	OBJ: exam spec C.III.G	TOP: image evaluation
83. **ANS: C**	REF: Ch. 7	OBJ: exam spec C.III.D	TOP: image evaxion
84. **ANS: A**	REF: Ch. 21	OBJ: exam spec C.III.E	TOP: image evaluation

85. **ANS: A**	REF: Ch. 10	OBJ: exam spec C.III.H	TOP: image evaluation
86. **ANS: B**	REF: Ch. 22	OBJ: exam spec D.I.A.2	TOP: ethics/legal issues
87. **ANS: A**	REF: Ch. 22	OBJ: exam spec D.I.A.1	TOP: ethics/legal issues
88. **ANS: C**	REF: Ch. 22	OBJ: exam spec D.I.B.3	TOP: ethics/legal issues
89. **ANS: B**	REF: Ch. 22	OBJ: exam spec D.II.A.1	TOP: interpersonal communications
90. **ANS: C**	REF: Ch. 22	OBJ: exam spec D.II.B.1	TOP: interpersonal communications
91. **ANS: B**	REF: Ch. 23	OBJ: exam spec D.IV.A	TOP: body mechanics
92. **ANS: A**	REF: Ch. 23	OBJ: exam spec D.III.B.4.d	TOP: infection control
93. **ANS: C**	REF: Ch. 23	OBJ: exam spec D.III.A.2.a	TOP: infection control
94. **ANS: D**	REF: Ch. 23	OBJ: exam spec D.III.C	TOP: infection control
95. **ANS: B**	REF: Ch. 23	OBJ: exam spec D.III.A.1	TOP: infection control
96. **ANS: A**	REF: Ch. 23	OBJ: exam spec D.III.C.1	TOP: infection control
97. **ANS: A**	REF: Ch. 23	OBJ: exam spec D.III.E.1	TOP: infection control
98. **ANS: B**	REF: Ch. 24	OBJ: exam spec D.V.A	TOP: medical emergencies
99. **ANS: D**	REF: Ch. 24	OBJ: exam spec D.V.C	TOP: medical emergencies
100. **ANS: D**	REF: Ch. 24	OBJ: exam spec D.IV.C.2	TOP: patient monitoring

Simulated Examination for the Limited Scope of Practice in Radiography—Chest Module

Complete this examination in pencil if you plan to take it more than once. If you are not sure of the answer to a question, skip it and return to it after completing the entire examination.

Multiple Choice

Identify the choice that best completes the statement or answers the question.

_____ 1. Refer to the diagram. What is the projection?

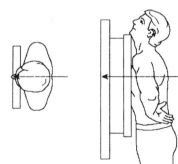

   A. Tangential
   B. Lateral
   C. Posteroanterior (PA)
   D. Anteroposterior (AP)

_____ 2. What structure separates the thoracic cavity from the abdominal cavity?
   A. The aortic arch
   B. The parietal membrane
   C. The visceral membrane
   D. The diaphragm

_____ 3. Which of the following organs are found within the mediastinum?
      1. Lungs
      2. Heart
      3. Trachea
   A. 1 and 2 only
   B. 1 and 3 only
   C. 2 and 3 only
   D. 1, 2, and 3

_____ 4. Three lobes are present in which lung(s)?
   A. The right lung
   B. The left lung
   C. Both lungs

_____ 5. What is the name of the upper portion of the lung?
   A. Costophrenic recess
   B. Costovertebral angle
   C. Apex
   D. Base

_____ 6. The inferior lateral corners of the lungs, visible on a PA chest radiograph, are called the:
   A. hila.
   B. apices.
   C. cardiophrenic angles.
   D. costophrenic angles.

_____ 7. When taking a PA projection of the chest, the recommended SID is:
   A. 30 inches.
   B. 40 inches.
   C. 60 inches.
   D. 72 inches.

____ 8. What is the purpose of the 72-inch SID used for chest radiography?
   A. Allows more room for accurate patient positioning
   B. Reduces patient dose
   C. Minimizes magnification of the heart shadow
   D. Minimizes demonstration of the scapula in the lungs

____ 9. Which of the following describe the importance of using an upright position for chest radiography?
   1. The upright position demonstrates air-fluid levels.
   2. The upright position allows maximum lung expansion.
   3. The upright position minimizes magnification of the heart.
   A. 1 and 2 only
   B. 1 and 3 only
   C. 2 and 3 only
   D. 1, 2, and 3

____ 10. In chest radiography, which body habitus is best imaged by placing the 35 × 43 cm IR crosswise in the upright grid cabinet?
   A. Sthenic
   B. Asthenic
   C. Hyposthenic
   D. Hypersthenic

____ 11. Which of the following techniques is desirable for chest radiography?
   A. High kVp, high mA, and short exposure time
   B. Low kVp and 40-inch SID
   C. Low kVp, long exposure time, and "breathing technique"
   D. High mAs and low kVp

____ 12. What is the purpose of rotating the patient's shoulders anteriorly for the PA projection of the chest?
   A. This motion rotates the scapulae out of the lungs.
   B. This motion reduces magnification of the heart shadow.
   C. This motion makes the position more comfortable for the patient.
   D. This motion places the coronal plane parallel to the upright grid cabinet.

____ 13. Where does the central ray enter the patient for the upright, PA projection of the chest?
   A. Midsagittal plane at the level of T7
   B. Midcoronal plane at the level of T7
   C. Midsagittal plane at the level of the iliac crests
   D. Midcoronal plane at the level of the iliac crests

____ 14. What is the proper placement of the arms for the upright lateral projection of the chest?
   A. Backs of the hands on the hips with the shoulders rolled anteriorly
   B. Arms raised over the head, hands grasping opposite elbows
   C. Arms abducted from thorax
   D. Arms adducted from thorax

____ 15. What are the proper patient instructions for the PA projection of the chest?
   A. Stop breathing after second deep inspiration.
   B. Stop breathing after deep inspiration.
   C. Stop breathing after expiration.
   D. Breath slowly and evenly.

____ 16. Lateral projections of the chest are taken with the left side against the IR because:
   A. lung pathology is more common on the left side.
   B. it is conventional to have a routine standard, and the left has been established as the standard.
   C. magnification of the cardiac silhouette is reduced with the left side nearer the IR.
   D. the right hilum provides high-contrast details that may be confusing.

____ 17. How much should the central ray be angled cephalad for an AP axial projection of the chest if the patient cannot assume the lordotic position?
   A. No angle is needed
   B. 10 degrees
   C. 15 degrees
   D. 25 degrees

____ 18. Which chest projection and position are needed to demonstrate free pleural fluid along the dependent chest wall?
   A. AP, upright
   B. PA, recumbent
   C. AP, lordotic
   D. AP, lateral decubitus

____ 19. Which of the following projections is best for demonstration of the apices of the lungs without bony superimposition?
   A. PA
   B. Lateral
   C. AP axial, lordotic position
   D. PA oblique

____ 20. Why is a grid used for routine chest radiography?
   A. To reduce scatter fog caused by use of high kVp
   B. To reduce patient dose by filtration
   C. To reduce magnification caused by increased SID
   D. To increase recorded detail

Simulated Examination for the Limited Scope of Practice in Radiography—Chest Module

Answer Section

Multiple Choice

1. **ANS: C**	REF: Ch. 14	OBJ: exam spec E.I.A.1	TOP: routine chest positioning
2. **ANS: D**	REF: Ch. 18	OBJ: exam spec E.I.A.2	TOP: chest anatomy
3. **ANS: C**	REF: Ch. 18	OBJ: exam spec E.I.A.2	TOP: chest anatomy
4. **ANS: A**	REF: Ch. 18	OBJ: exam spec E.I.A.2	TOP: chest anatomy
5. **ANS: C**	REF: Ch. 18	OBJ: exam spec E.I.A.2	TOP: chest anatomy
6. **ANS: D**	REF: Ch. 18	OBJ: exam spec E.I.A.2	TOP: chest anatomy
7. **ANS: D**	REF: Ch. 18	OBJ: exam spec E.I.A.1	TOP: routine chest positioning
8. **ANS: C**	REF: Ch. 18	OBJ: exam spec E.I.A.1	TOP: routine chest positioning
9. **ANS: D**	REF: Ch. 18	OBJ: exam spec E.I.A.1	TOP: routine chest positioning
10. **ANS: D**	REF: Ch. 18	OBJ: exam spec E.I.A.1	TOP: routine chest positioning
11. **ANS: A**	REF: Ch. 18	OBJ: exam spec E.I.A.3	TOP: routine chest technical factors
12. **ANS: A**	REF: Ch. 18	OBJ: exam spec E.I.A.1	TOP: routine chest positioning
13. **ANS: A**	REF: Ch. 18	OBJ: exam spec E.I.A.1	TOP: routine chest positioning
14. **ANS: B**	REF: Ch. 18	OBJ: exam spec E.I.A.1	TOP: routine chest positioning
15. **ANS: A**	REF: Ch. 18	OBJ: exam spec E.I.A.1	TOP: routine chest positioning
16. **ANS: C**	REF: Ch. 18	OBJ: exam spec E.I.A.1	TOP: routine chest positioning
17. **ANS: C**	REF: Ch. 18	OBJ: exam spec E.I.B.1	TOP: other chest positioning
18. **ANS: D**	REF: Ch. 18	OBJ: exam spec E.I.B.1	TOP: other chest positioning
19. **ANS: C**	REF: Ch. 18	OBJ: exam spec E.I.B.1	TOP: other chest positioning
20. **ANS: A**	REF: Ch. 18	OBJ: exam spec E.I.A.4	TOP: routine chest equipment

Simulated Examination for the Limited Scope of Practice in Radiography—Extremities Module

Complete this examination in pencil if you plan to take it more than once. If you are not sure of the answer to a question, skip it and return to it after completing the entire examination.

Multiple Choice

Identify the choice that best completes the statement or answers the question.

____ 1. Which of the following bones are in the hindfoot portion of the foot?
   1. Cuneiforms
   2. Calcaneus
   3. Talus
   A. 1 and 2 only
   B. 1 and 3 only
   C. 2 and 3 only
   D. 1, 2, and 3

_____ 2. The anatomic name for the bone commonly known as the *kneecap* is the:
   A. fibula.
   B. tibia.
   C. patella.
   D. fabella.

_____ 3. The palpable portion at the distal end of the tibia is called the:
   A. lateral malleolus.
   B. medial malleolus.
   C. medial condyle.
   D. lateral condyle.

_____ 4. When the ankle is flexed to raise the foot, the movement is termed:
   A. plantar flexion.
   B. eversion.
   C. inversion.
   D. dorsiflexion.

_____ 5. What device may help provide an even density on a radiograph of an anteroposterior (AP) axial projection of the foot?
   A. Lead shield
   B. Wedge compensating filter
   C. Wedge positioning sponge
   D. Sandbag

_____ 6. Which of the following is true regarding the correct positioning of the ankle for a lateral projection?
   A. The medial surface of the ankle joint is in contact with the IR.
   B. The sagittal plane of the foot and leg is perpendicular to the IR.
   C. The central ray enters perpendicular to the medial malleolus.
   D. The ankle joint is extended so that the foot is 15 to 20 degrees from the IR.

_____ 7. When the leg is extended in the supine position, the ankle is maximally dorsiflexed, and the central ray is directed 40 degrees cephalad through the plantar surface of the foot, the resulting image will demonstrate:
   A. an axial projection of the calcaneus.
   B. a medial oblique position of the tarsals and metatarsals.
   C. the ankle mortise, especially the talofibular articulation.
   D. the cuboid and the third cuneiform.

_____ 8. Which of the following are true regarding the correct position for an AP projection of the lower leg?
   1. The leg should be extended and resting on the IR.
   2. The ankle should be dorsiflexed so that the foot forms a 90-degree angle with the lower leg.
   3. The sagittal plane of the leg is placed parallel to the IR.
   A. 1 and 2 only
   B. 1 and 3 only
   C. 2 and 3 only
   D. 1, 2, and 3

_____ 9. Where should the central ray enter the patient for the AP projection of the knee?
   A. ½ inch below the apex of the patella
   B. ½ inch below the base of the patella
   C. 1 inch distal to the medial epicondyle of the femur
   D. 1 inch proximal to the medial epicondyle of the femur

_____ 10. When a lateral projection of the knee is taken, flexion of the knee joint should be limited to 10 degrees when there is suspicion of:
   A. a loose fragment within the joint.
   B. collateral ligament injury.
   C. damage to the medial meniscus cartilage.
   D. a fracture of the patella.

_____ 11. What change in technical factors is required when an ankle in a dry plaster cast must be radiographed?
   A. Increase mAs by 2 times
   C. Decrease mAs by ½
   B. Increase mAs by 3 times
   D. Decrease mAs by ¼

_____ 12. The bones that are located in the palm of the hand are called:
   A. carpals.
   B. phalanges.
   C. metacarpals.
   D. digits.

_____ 13. The bones of the forearm are the:
   A. radius and ulna.
   B. tibia and fibula.
   C. humerus and radius.
   D. clavicle and scapula.

_____ 14. Where is the humerus located?
A. At the anterior portion of the shoulder girdle
B. At the posterior portion of the shoulder girdle
C. On the lateral side of the forearm
D. In the upper portion of the arm

_____ 15. Which surface of the hand should be in contact with the IR for the posteroanterior (PA) projection?
A. Lateral
B. Medial
C. Posterior (dorsal)
D. Anterior (palmar)

_____ 16. What is the center point of the central ray for the PA projection of the hand?
A. Third metacarpophalangeal joint
B. Second metacarpophalangeal joint
C. Third proximal interphalangeal joint
D. Base of the third metacarpal

_____ 17. Which surface of the hand should be in contact with the IR for the lateral projection of the fifth digit (pinky)?
A. The medial surface
B. The lateral surface
C. The anterior (palmar) surface
D. The posterior (dorsal) surface

_____ 18. What is the position of the wrist for the PA oblique projection in lateral rotation?
A. Hand and wrist flat with anterior surface in contact with IR
B. Fingers flexed with anterior surface of wrist in contact with IR
C. Coronal plane of wrist at 45-degree angle to IR with anteromedial surface on IR
D. Medial surface of wrist on IR with coronal plane perpendicular to IR

_____ 19. What is the proper patient position for the AP projection of the forearm?
A. Elbow extended, wrist and elbow parallel to IR, hand supinated
B. Elbow extended, wrist and elbow parallel to IR, hand pronated
C. Elbow flexed, wrist and elbow perpendicular to IR, hand in lateral position
D. Elbow flexed, wrist and elbow perpendicular to IR, hand pronated

_____ 20. Which of the following describes the proper method to position the humerus for an AP projection?
A. Upper limb adducted, elbow flexed, humeral epicondyles perpendicular to IR
B. Upper limb abducted, elbow extended, humeral epicondyles parallel to IR
C. Upper limb adducted, elbow extended, humeral epicondyles parallel to IR
D. Upper limb abducted, elbow flexed, humeral epicondyles perpendicular to IR

_____ 21. What specific anatomy is demonstrated without superimposition in the AP oblique projection in 45-degree lateral rotation?
A. Radial head and capitulum
B. Superimposed humeral epicondyles and open elbow joint
C. Olecranon process in profile
D. Coronoid process of the ulna and the trochlea

_____ 22. What change in technical factors is required when a wrist in a fiberglass cast must be radiographed?
A. No change is required.
C. Increase mAs by 3 times.
B. Increase mAs by 2 times.
D. Decrease mAs by ¼.

_____ 23. Where is the central ray entrance point for the AP projections of the shoulder?
A. 1 inch superior to the coracoid process
B. 1 inch medial and inferior to the coracoid process
C. 1 inch medial and inferior to the acromion
D. 1 inch superior to the acromion

_____ 24. What are the proper patient instructions for the AP projection of the shoulder?
A. Stop breathing and do not move.
B. Breathe quietly and do not move.
C. Take slow, deep breaths and do not move.
D. Pant quickly and do not move.

_____ 25. What is the name of the large, rounded projection that can be felt on the superior lateral surface of the shoulder?
A. Coracoid process
B. Lateral epicondyle
C. Acromion
D. Inferior angle of the scapula

Simulated Examination for the Limited Scope of Practice in Radiography—Extremities Module

Answer Section

Multiple Choice

1. **ANS: C**	REF: Ch. 16	OBJ: exam spec E.II.A.2	TOP: lower extremity anatomy
2. **ANS: C**	REF: Ch. 16	OBJ: exam spec E.II.A.2	TOP: lower extremity anatomy
3. **ANS: B**	REF: Ch. 16	OBJ: exam spec E.II.A.2	TOP: lower extremity anatomy
4. **ANS: D**	REF: Ch. 16	OBJ: exam spec E.II.A.1	TOP: lower extremity positioning
5. **ANS: B**	REF: Ch. 16	OBJ: exam spec E.II.A.4	TOP: lower extremity accessory equipment
6. **ANS: C**	REF: Ch. 16	OBJ: exam spec E.II.A.1	TOP: lower extremity positioning
7. **ANS: A**	REF: Ch. 16	OBJ: exam spec E.II.A.1	TOP: lower extremity positioning
8. **ANS: A**	REF: Ch. 16	OBJ: exam spec E.II.A.1	TOP: lower extremity positioning
9. **ANS: A**	REF: Ch. 16	OBJ: exam spec E.II.A.1	TOP: lower extremity positioning
10. **ANS: D**	REF: Ch. 16	OBJ: exam spec E.II.A.1	TOP: lower extremity positioning
11. **ANS: A**	REF: Ch. 12	OBJ: exam spec E.II.A.3	TOP: lower extremity technical factors
12. **ANS: C**	REF: Ch. 15	OBJ: exam spec E.II.B.2	TOP: upper extremity anatomy
13. **ANS: A**	REF: Ch. 15	OBJ: exam spec E.II.B.2	TOP: upper extremity anatomy
14. **ANS: D**	REF: Ch. 15	OBJ: exam spec E.II.B.2	TOP: upper extremity anatomy
15. **ANS: D**	REF: Ch. 15	OBJ: exam spec E.II.B.1	TOP: upper extremity positioning
16. **ANS: A**	REF: Ch. 15	OBJ: exam spec E.II.B.1	TOP: upper extremity positioning
17. **ANS: A**	REF: Ch. 15	OBJ: exam spec E.II.B.1	TOP: upper extremity positioning
18. **ANS: C**	REF: Ch. 15	OBJ: exam spec E.II.B.1	TOP: upper extremity positioning
19. **ANS: A**	REF: Ch. 15	OBJ: exam spec E.II.B.1	TOP: upper extremity positioning
20. **ANS: B**	REF: Ch. 15	OBJ: exam spec E.II.B.1	TOP: upper extremity positioning
21. **ANS: A**	REF: Ch. 15	OBJ: exam spec E.II.B.1	TOP: upper extremity positioning
22. **ANS: A**	REF: Ch. 12	OBJ: exam spec E.II.B.3	TOP: upper extremity technical factors
23. **ANS: B**	REF: Ch. 15	OBJ: exam spec E.II.C.1	TOP: shoulder positioning
24. **ANS: A**	REF: Ch. 15	OBJ: exam spec E.II.C.1	TOP: shoulder positioning
25. **ANS: C**	REF: Ch. 15	OBJ: exam spec E.II.C.2	TOP: shoulder anatomy

Simulated Examination for the Limited Scope of Practice in Radiography—Skull/Sinuses Module

Complete this examination in pencil if you plan to take it more than once. If you are not sure of the answer to a question, skip it and return to it after completing the entire examination.

Multiple Choice

Identify the choice that best completes the statement or answers the question.

_____ 1. Which of the following cranial bones are paired (right and left)?
  1. Frontal
  2. Parietal
  3. Temporal
  A. 1 only
  B. 1 and 2 only
  C. 2 and 3 only
  D. 1, 2, and 3

_____ 2. What structure serves as the passageway for the spinal cord to exit the skull and pass into the spinal canal of the vertebral column?
  A. External auditory meatus (EAM)
  B. Foramen magnum
  C. Sella turcica
  D. Crista galli

_____ 3. When taking a posteroanterior (PA) axial projection (Caldwell method) of the skull, the central ray is directed:
  A. 15 degrees cephalad.
  B. 15 degrees caudad.
  C. 30 degrees cephalad.
  D. 30 degrees caudad.

_____ 4. Which radiographic baseline is used to position the PA axial projection (Caldwell method) of the cranium?
  A. Either the OML or the IOML can be used
  B. Mentomeatal line
  C. IOML
  D. OML

_____ 5. Which cranial projection best demonstrates the occipital bone?
A. Posteroanterior (PA)
B. PA axial (Caldwell method)
C. Anteroposterior (AP) axial (Towne method)
D. Lateral

_____ 6. The patient is in a prone oblique position with the midsagittal plane of the head parallel to the IR and the interpupillary line perpendicular to the IR. The central ray is directed perpendicularly to enter 2 inches superior to the EAM. What projection of the cranium will be demonstrated on the radiograph?
A. Lateral
B. AP axial (Towne method)
C. PA axial (Caldwell method)
D. PA

_____ 7. The patient is positioned supine with the midsagittal plane and OML perpendicular to the IR. The central ray is angled 30 degrees caudad and enters the midsagittal plane at approximately 2.5 inches superior to the glabella. What projection will be imaged on the radiograph?
A. Lateral
B. PA axial (Caldwell method)
C. PA
D. AP axial (Towne method)

_____ 8. What positioning accessory can be used to assist the patient in holding the correct position for an AP axial projection of the skull?
A. A lead mask
C. A wedge sponge
B. A wedge filter
D. An angiligner

_____ 9. Air-filled cavities located in some bones of the face and cranium are called:
A. cranial sutures.
B. zygomatic prominences.
C. paranasal sinuses.
D. paranasal foramina.

_____ 10. Which of the following bones contain paranasal sinuses?
1. Frontal
2. Ethmoid
3. Temporal
A. 1 and 2 only
B. 1 and 3 only
C. 2 and 3 only
D. 1, 2, and 3

_____ 11. What is the purpose of performing sinus radiography with the patient in the upright position?
A. To demonstrate air/fluid levels
B. For ease of patient positioning
C. To prevent superimposition of the cranial structures on the paranasal sinuses
D. Sinus radiography does not have to be performed with the patient upright

_____ 12. Which paranasal sinuses are best demonstrated in the PA axial projection (Caldwell method)?
1. Maxillary
2. Frontal
3. Ethmoid
A. 1 and 2 only
B. 1 and 3 only
C. 2 and 3 only
D. 1, 2, and 3

_____ 13. Which of the following projections will demonstrate the sphenoid sinus?
A. Parietoacanthial (Waters method)
B. Lateral
C. AP axial (Towne method)
D. PA axial (Caldwell method)

_____ 14. Which projection best demonstrates the maxillary sinuses?
A. Parietoacanthial (Waters method)
B. SMV
C. PA axial (Caldwell method)
D. AP axial (Towne method)

_____ 15. Which paranasal sinuses are demonstrated by the SMV projection?
1. Sphenoid
2. Ethmoid
3. Maxillary
A. 1 and 2 only
B. 1 and 3 only
C. 2 and 3 only
D. 1, 2, and 3

_____ 16. Which projection will demonstrate all of the paranasal sinuses?
A. PA axial (Caldwell method)
B. Parietoacanthial (Waters method)
C. Lateral
D. SMV

_____ 17. What is the medical term for the bony sockets that house the eyes?
A. Eye sockets
B. Supraorbital margins
C. Glabella
D. Orbits

____ 18. A lateral projection of the face using detail screens tabletop (nongrid) is used to demonstrate the:
A. mandible.
B. zygoma.
C. orbits.
D. nasal bones.

____ 19. Which projection of the facial bones requires the central ray to exit the acanthion?
A. AP axial (Towne method)
B. PA axial (Caldwell method)
C. Lateral
D. Parietoacanthial (Waters method)

____ 20. What is the proper central ray angle and direction for the axiolateral projection of the mandible when the midsagittal plane of the head is angled 15 degrees toward the IR?
A. 10 degrees cephalad
B. 10 degrees caudad
C. 25 degrees cephalad
D. 25 degrees caudad

Simulated Examination for the Limited Scope of Practice in Radiography—Skull/Sinuses Module

Answer Section

Multiple Choice

1. **ANS: C**	REF: Ch. 19	OBJ: exam spec E.III.A.2	TOP: skull anatomy
2. **ANS: B**	REF: Ch. 19	OBJ: exam spec E.III.A.2	TOP: skull anatomy
3. **ANS: B**	REF: Ch. 19	OBJ: exam spec E.III.A.2	TOP: skull anatomy
4. **ANS: D**	REF: Ch. 19	OBJ: exam spec E.III.A.1	TOP: skull positioning
5. **ANS: C**	REF: Ch. 19	OBJ: exam spec E.III.A.1	TOP: skull positioning
6. **ANS: A**	REF: Ch. 19	OBJ: exam spec E.III.A.1	TOP: skull positioning
7. **ANS: D**	REF: Ch. 19	OBJ: exam spec E.III.A.1	TOP: skull positioning
8. **ANS: C**	REF: Ch. 19	OBJ: exam spec E.III.A.4	TOP: skull positioning accessory
9. **ANS: C**	REF: Ch. 19	OBJ: exam spec E.III.B.2	TOP: sinus anatomy
10. **ANS: A**	REF: Ch. 19	OBJ: exam spec E.III.B.2	TOP: sinus anatomy
11. **ANS: A**	REF: Ch. 19	OBJ: exam spec E.III.B.3	TOP: sinus technique
12. **ANS: C**	REF: Ch. 19	OBJ: exam spec E.III.B.1	TOP: sinus positioning
13. **ANS: B**	REF: Ch. 19	OBJ: exam spec E.III.B.1	TOP: sinus positioning
14. **ANS: A**	REF: Ch. 19	OBJ: exam spec E.III.B.1	TOP: sinus positioning
15. **ANS: A**	REF: Ch. 19	OBJ: exam spec E.III.B.1	TOP: sinus positioning
16. **ANS: C**	REF: Ch. 19	OBJ: exam spec E.III.B.1	TOP: sinus positioning
17. **ANS: D**	REF: Ch. 19	OBJ: exam spec E.III.C.2	TOP: facial bones anatomy
18. **ANS: D**	REF: Ch. 19	OBJ: exam spec E.III.C.1	TOP: facial bones positioning
19. **ANS: D**	REF: Ch. 19	OBJ: exam spec E.III.C.1	TOP: facial bones positioning
20. **ANS: A**	REF: Ch. 19	OBJ: exam spec E.III.C.1	TOP: facial bones positioning

Simulated Examination for the Limited Scope of Practice in Radiography—Spine Module

Complete this examination in pencil if you plan to take it more than once. If you are not sure of the answer to a question, skip it and return to it after completing the entire examination.

Multiple Choice

Identify the choice that best completes the statement or answers the question.

____ 1. How many vertebrae are located in the cervical region of the spine?
A. 5
B. 12
C. 7
D. 9

____ 2. What is the odontoid process and where is it located?
   A. A sharp process on the inferior surface of C1
   B. A toothlike projection on the superior surface of C2
   C. A rounded prominence on the posterior aspect of C7
   D. A palpable landmark on the mandible

____ 3. When taking an anteroposterior (AP) axial projection of the cervical spine, the central ray is directed:
   A. 15 degrees caudad.
   B. 15 degrees cephalad.
   C. 25 degrees caudad.
   D. 25 degrees cephalad.

____ 4. What is the rationale for using a 72-inch SID for the lateral projection of the cervical spine?
   A. This SID enables the limited operator to use a lower-kVp technique.
   B. This SID reduces patient dose.
   C. This SID helps to overcome the magnification caused by the increased OID of the position.
   D. This SID provides more room for the limited operator to assist the patient into the proper position.

____ 5. What anatomic structures of the cervical spine are best demonstrated by the lateral projection?
   A. Intervertebral discs
   B. Intervertebral foramina
   C. Zygapophyseal joints
   D. Pedicles

____ 6. What is the proper central ray angle and direction for the AP oblique projections of the cervical spine?
   A. 15 degrees cephalad
   B. 15 degrees caudad
   C. 45 degrees cephalad
   D. 45 degrees caudad

____ 7. What is the proper patient position for an AP oblique projection of the cervical spine?
   A. 45-degree posterior oblique position
   B. 45-degree anterior oblique position
   C. Coronal plane positioned parallel to the IR
   D. Supine with the base of the skull aligned with the edge of the front teeth

____ 8. What anatomic structures are best demonstrated by the posteroanterior (PA) oblique projections of the cervical spine?
   A. Zygapophyseal joints closer to the IR
   B. Zygapophyseal joints farther from the IR
   C. Intervertebral foramina closer to the IR
   D. Intervertebral foramina farther from the IR

____ 9. How many vertebrae comprise the thoracic spine?
   A. 5
   B. 7
   C. 12
   D. 22

____ 10. Which vertebrae have special facets for articulation with the ribs?
   A. Cervical
   B. Thoracic
   C. Lumbar
   D. Sacral

____ 11. Breathing technique is used to advantage when taking a lateral projection of the:
   A. cervical spine.
   B. thoracic spine.
   C. lumbar spine.
   D. sacrum.

____ 12. The patient is positioned with the coronal plane of the body perpendicular to the IR, the midsagittal plane parallel to the IR, and the arm closest to the IR raised over the head. The central ray is perpendicular and centered to the level of the C7-T1 interspace. What projection and anatomy will be demonstrated in this image?
   A. A lateral projection of the cervicothoracic region
   B. An AP projection of the lower cervical spine
   C. A lateral projection of the lower cervical spine
   D. An AP projection of the cervicothoracic region

____ 13. What device(s) may be used to improve visualization of the spinous processes of the thoracic spine on the lateral projection?
   A. A piece of lead placed behind the shadow of the patient's back
   B. A wedge filter placed with the thicker end on the upper thoracic spine
   C. A sandbag placed near the patient's shoulders and another put near the patient's hips
   D. A positioning sponge used to elevate the patient's waist

____ 14. Which structures should be seen on the lateral projection of the thoracic spine?
   A. C7 through L1
   B. T3 through T12
   C. C5 through T7
   D. C6 through L2

____ 15. What is the number of vertebrae in the normal lumbar spine?
   A. 4
   B. 5
   C. 7
   D. 8

____ 16. Which portion of the spine is made up of five vertebrae and has a lordotic curve?
   A. Cervical
   B. Thoracic
   C. Lumbar
   D. Sacrum

____ 17. When using a 35 × 43 cm IR, where should the central ray enter the patient for an AP projection of the lumbar spine?
   A. At the level of the iliac crest in the midline of the patient
   B. At a level 1½ inches superior to the iliac crest in the midline of the patient
   C. At the level of the sacrum along the coronal plane of the patient
   D. This size IR is not appropriate for lumbar spine images

____ 18. When using a 30 × 35 cm IR, where should the central ray enter the patient for an AP projection of the lumbar spine?
   A. At the level of the iliac crest in the midline of the patient
   B. At a level 1½ inches superior to the iliac crest in the midline of the patient
   C. At the level of the sacrum along the coronal plane of the patient
   D. This size IR is not appropriate for lumbar spine images

____ 19. What positioning maneuver is used to improve patient comfort and reduce the lordotic curve of the lumbar spine when positioning a recumbent patient for an AP projection of the lumbar spine?
   A. Raising the patient's arms above the head
   B. Crossing the patient's arms across the chest
   C. Flexing the knees and using a support under them
   D. Having the patient distribute weight equally on both feet

____ 20. Which projection of the lumbar spine demonstrates open intervertebral foramina?
   A. AP
   B. PA
   C. Lateral
   D. AP oblique

____ 21. Which of the following body positions will demonstrate the left zygapophyseal joints of the lumbar spine?
   A. Left lateral
   B. 45 degrees RPO
   C. 45 degrees LAO
   D. 45 degrees LPO

____ 22. What specific anatomy is best demonstrated on the AP oblique projection of the lumbar spine if the patient is positioned in a 45-degree RPO position?
   A. Right intervertebral foramina
   B. Right zygapophyseal joints
   C. Left intervertebral foramina
   D. Left zygapophyseal joints

____ 23. What is the central ray angle and direction for the AP axial projection of the sacrum?
   A. 10 degrees cephalad
   B. 10 degrees caudad
   C. 15 degrees cephalad
   D. 15 degrees caudad

____ 24. What portion of the spine is commonly call the *tail bone?*
   A. Thoracic spine
   B. Lumbar spine
   C. Sacrum
   D. Coccyx

____ 25. Which of the following statements is *true* regarding spine radiography to evaluate scoliosis?
   A. The AP projection is preferred.
   B. No patient shielding should be used.
   C. The IR should extend from the top of the patient's ear to the level of the greater trochanter.
   D. A 30-inch SID is recommended.

Simulated Examination for the Limited Scope of Practice in Radiography—Spine Module

Answer Section

Multiple Choice

1. ANS: C	REF: Ch. 17	OBJ: exam spec E.IV.A.2	TOP: cervical spine anatomy
2. ANS: B	REF: Ch. 17	OBJ: exam spec E.IV.A.2	TOP: cervical spine anatomy
3. ANS: B	REF: Ch. 17	OBJ: exam spec E.IV.A.1	TOP: cervical spine positioning
4. ANS: C	REF: Ch. 17	OBJ: exam spec E.IV.A.3	TOP: cervical spine technique
5. ANS: C	REF: Ch. 17	OBJ: exam spec E.IV.A.1	TOP: cervical spine positioning
6. ANS: A	REF: Ch. 17	OBJ: exam spec E.IV.A.1	TOP: cervical spine positioning
7. ANS: A	REF: Ch. 17	OBJ: exam spec E.IV.A.1	TOP: cervical spine positioning
8. ANS: C	REF: Ch. 17	OBJ: exam spec E.IV.A.1	TOP: cervical spine positioning
9. ANS: C	REF: Ch. 17	OBJ: exam spec E.IV.B.2	TOP: thoracic spine anatomy
10. ANS: B	REF: Ch. 17	OBJ: exam spec E.IV.B.2	TOP: thoracic spine anatomy
11. ANS: B	REF: Ch. 17	OBJ: exam spec E.IV.B.1	TOP: thoracic spine positioning
12. ANS: A	REF: Ch. 17	OBJ: exam spec E.IV.B.1	TOP: thoracic spine positioning
13. ANS: A	REF: Ch. 17	OBJ: exam spec E.IV.B.4	TOP: thoracic spine positioning accessories
14. ANS: B	REF: Ch. 17	OBJ: exam spec E.IV.B.1	TOP: thoracic spine positioning
15. ANS: B	REF: Ch. 17	OBJ: exam spec E.IV.C.2	TOP: lumbar spine anatomy
16. ANS: C	REF: Ch. 17	OBJ: exam spec E.IV.C.2	TOP: lumbar spine anatomy
17. ANS: A	REF: Ch. 17	OBJ: exam spec E.IV.C.1	TOP: lumbar spine positioning
18. ANS: B	REF: Ch. 17	OBJ: exam spec E.IV.C.1	TOP: lumbar spine positioning
19. ANS: C	REF: Ch. 17	OBJ: exam spec E.IV.C.1	TOP: lumbar spine positioning
20. ANS: C	REF: Ch. 17	OBJ: exam spec E.IV.C.1	TOP: lumbar spine positioning
21. ANS: D	REF: Ch. 17	OBJ: exam spec E.IV.C.1	TOP: lumbar spine positioning
22. ANS: B	REF: Ch. 17	OBJ: exam spec E.IV.C.1	TOP: lumbar spine positioning
23. ANS: C	REF: Ch. 17	OBJ: exam spec E.IV.D.1	TOP: sacrum positioning
24. ANS: D	REF: Ch. 17	OBJ: exam spec E.IV.D.2	TOP: coccyx anatomy
25. ANS: C	REF: Ch. 17	OBJ: exam spec E.IV.E.1	TOP: scoliosis spine positioning

Simulated Examination for the Limited Scope of Practice in Radiography—Podiatry Module

Complete this examination in pencil if you plan to take it more than once. If you are not sure of the answer to a question, skip it and return to it after completing the entire examination.

Multiple Choice

Identify the choice that best completes the statement or answers the question.

_____ 1. The bones of the forefoot include the:
A. phalanges and tarsals.
B. tarsals and metatarsals.
C. phalanges and metatarsals.
D. cuneiforms and cuboid.

_____ 2. The bones of the midfoot are called the:
A. metatarsals.
B. tarsals.
C. phalanges.
D. cuneiforms.

_____ 3. Small, flat, oval bones in the region of the first metatarsophalangeal joint are called the:
A. phalanges.
B. tarsals.
C. metatarsals.
D. sesamoid bones.

_____ 4. What tarsal is commonly referred to as the *heel bone*?
A. Talus
B. Cuneiforms
C. Navicular
D. Calcaneus

_____ 5. Which of the following bones are tarsal bones?
1. Cuneiforms
2. Cuboid
3. Calcaneus
A. 1 and 2 only
B. 1 and 3 only
C. 2 and 3 only
D. 1, 2, and 3

_____ 6. When taking an anteroposterior (AP) axial projection of the foot, the central ray is directed:
A. 10 degrees toward the toes.
B. 10 degrees toward the heel.
C. 25 degrees toward the heel.
D. perpendicular to the IR.

_____ 7. Where does the central ray enter the patient for the AP axial projection of the foot?
A. At the third metatarsophalangeal (MTP) joint
B. At the first MTP joint
C. At the base of the third metatarsal
D. At the head of the third metatarsal

_____ 8. Which surface of the foot should be in contact with the IR for the lateral projection of the foot?
A. Lateral
B. Medial
C. Dorsal
D. Plantar

_____ 9. Which of the following is true regarding the lateral projection of the foot?
A. The ankle does not have a specific position when a lateral projection of the foot is performed.
B. The ankle should be dorsiflexed so that the long axis of the foot forms a 45-degree angle with the tibia.
C. The ankle should be extended so that the plantar surface of the foot forms a 45-degree angle with the IR.
D. The ankle should be dorsiflexed so that the long axis of the foot is perpendicular to the tibia.

_____ 10. How much is the plantar surface of the foot elevated from the IR for the AP oblique projection of the foot?
A. 45 degrees
B. 30 degrees
C. 10 degrees
D. 25 degrees

_____ 11. Which foot projection and position will demonstrate the metatarsals (third through fifth) without superimposition?
A. AP axial projection with the plantar surface of the foot in contact with the IR
B. AP oblique projection in 30-degree lateral rotation
C. AP oblique projection in 30-degree medial rotation
D. Lateral projection with the MTP joints perpendicular to the IR

_____ 12. Which foot projection and position will demonstrate the medial and intermediate cuneiforms without superimposition?
A. AP axial projection with the plantar surface of the foot in contact with the IR
B. AP oblique projection in 30-degree lateral rotation
C. AP oblique projection in 30-degree medial rotation
D. Lateral projection with the MTP joints perpendicular to the IR

_____ 13. Which foot projection and position will demonstrate the cuboid, navicular, and lateral cuneiforms without superimposition?
A. AP axial projection with the plantar surface of the foot in contact with the IR
B. AP oblique projection in 30-degree lateral rotation
C. AP oblique projection in 30-degree medial rotation
D. Lateral projection with the MTP joints perpendicular to the IR

_____ 14. Which foot projection and position will demonstrate the entire foot in near anatomic position?
A. AP axial projection with the plantar surface of the foot in contact with the IR
B. AP oblique projection in 30-degree lateral rotation
C. AP oblique projection in 30-degree medial rotation
D. Lateral projection with the MTP joints perpendicular to the IR

_____ 15. What is the name given to the distal end of the fibula?
A. Talus
B. Medial malleolus
C. Lateral malleolus
D. Astragalus

____ 16. Which of the following are the bones that articulate to form the ankle mortise?
A. Talus, tibia, and fibula
B. Tibia, fibula, and calcaneus
C. Talus and tibia
D. Calcaneus and tibia

____ 17. When the leg is extended, the ankle is dorsiflexed to form an angle of 90 degrees between foot and leg, the leg is rotated medially approximately 15 degrees, and the central ray is perpendicular to the IR through the midpoint between the malleoli, the resulting image will demonstrate:
A. an axial projection of the calcaneus.
B. an AP projection of the tarsals and metatarsals.
C. the ankle mortise, especially the talofibular articulation.
D. the cuboid and the third cuneiform.

____ 18. Where should the central ray enter the patient for the AP projection of the ankle joint?
A. Perpendicular to a point midway between the malleoli
B. Perpendicular to the base of the third metatarsal
C. Angled 10 degrees cephalad to a point midway between the malleoli
D. Angled 10 degrees cephalad to the base of the third metatarsal

____ 19. Which surface of the ankle is placed in contact with the IR for the lateral projection of the ankle?
A. Medial surface
B. Lateral surface
C. Anterior surface
D. Posterior surface

____ 20. What is the proper central ray angle and direction for the axial projection of the calcaneus when the ankle is dorsiflexed so that the plantar surface of the foot is perpendicular to the IR?
A. 10 degrees cephalad
B. 40 degrees cephalad
C. 10 degrees caudad
D. 40 degrees caudad

Simulated Examination for the Limited Scope of Practice in Radiography—Podiatry Module

Answer Section

Multiple Choice

1. **ANS: C**	REF: Ch. 16	OBJ: exam spec E.V.A.2	TOP: foot anatomy
2. **ANS: B**	REF: Ch. 16	OBJ: exam spec E.V.A.2	TOP: foot anatomy
3. **ANS: D**	REF: Ch. 16	OBJ: exam spec E.V.A.2	TOP: foot anatomy
4. **ANS: D**	REF: Ch. 16	OBJ: exam spec E.V.A.2	TOP: foot anatomy
5. **ANS: A**	REF: Ch. 16	OBJ: exam spec E.V.A.2	TOP: foot anatomy
6. **ANS: B**	REF: Ch. 16	OBJ: exam spec E.V.A.1	TOP: foot positioning
7. **ANS: C**	REF: Ch. 16	OBJ: exam spec E.V.A.1	TOP: foot positioning
8. **ANS: A**	REF: Ch. 16	OBJ: exam spec E.V.A.1	TOP: foot positioning
9. **ANS: D**	REF: Ch. 16	OBJ: exam spec E.V.A.1	TOP: foot positioning
10. **ANS: B**	REF: Ch. 16	OBJ: exam spec E.V.A.1	TOP: foot positioning
11. **ANS: C**	REF: Ch. 16	OBJ: exam spec E.V.A.1	TOP: foot positioning
12. **ANS: B**	REF: Ch. 16	OBJ: exam spec E.V.A.1	TOP: foot positioning
13. **ANS: C**	REF: Ch. 16	OBJ: exam spec E.V.A.1	TOP: foot positioning
14. **ANS: A**	REF: Ch. 16	OBJ: exam spec E.V.A.1	TOP: foot positioning
15. **ANS: C**	REF: Ch. 16	OBJ: exam spec E.V.B.2	TOP: ankle anatomy

16. **ANS: A**   REF: Ch. 16   OBJ: exam spec E.V.B.2   TOP: ankle anatomy
17. **ANS: C**   REF: Ch. 16   OBJ: exam spec E.V.B.1   TOP: ankle positioning
18. **ANS: A**   REF: Ch. 16   OBJ: exam spec E.V.B.1   TOP: ankle positioning
19. **ANS: B**   REF: Ch. 16   OBJ: exam spec E.V.B.1   TOP: ankle positioning
20. **ANS: B**   REF: Ch. 16   OBJ: exam spec E.V.C.1   TOP: calcaneus positioning

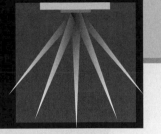

Preparation Guide for the American Registry of Radiologic Technologists Bone Densitometry Equipment Operators Examination

Introduction

This guide is provided to help you prepare to successfully complete the licensure exam for the limited scope of practice in bone densitometry. We have included helpful suggestions for optimizing your study time and a simulated examination to help you identify your areas of strength and weakness. All suggestions and discussion are based on the American Registry of Radiologic Technologists (ARRT) Content Specifications for the Bone Densitometry Equipment Operators Examination. We have done this for two reasons: first, this is a comprehensive examination covering all relevant areas of practice; and second, it is likely that the licensure agency in your state uses this examination. If your state does not use this examination you will still be well prepared if you use the ARRT Content Specifications as your study guide. For your convenience, we have included the most recent ARRT Content Specifications in this guide.

If you are using *Radiography Essentials for Limited Practice* and this accompanying workbook, it is likely that you are participating in an educational program designed to prepare you both to work in the practice area and to successfully pass the appropriate state licensure examination. This guide should assist you in both these endeavors. Completing the simulated examination will help you identify knowledge that you have already acquired and knowledge that you have yet to master. Since the simulated examination was constructed to assess content identified in the ARRT Content Specifications, it is appropriate to provide an overview of this document before moving on to the examination.

The ARRT Content Specifications for the Bone Densitometry Equipment Operators Examination covers eight content areas. These include basic concepts, equipment operation and quality control (QC), radiation safety, and dual energy x-ray absorptiometry (DXA) scanning of the finger, heel (os calcis or calcaneus), forearm, lumbar spine, and proximal femur. Although it is not likely that you will perform bone densitometry procedures on all five of these body parts, the ARRT philosophy is that you should be able to demonstrate a basic understanding of all these procedures to ensure your ability to perform any of the procedures. This is also in your best interest, because then you will not be limited to one area of bone densitometry practice.

The most valuable component of the Content Specifications is the outline of each content area covered on the examination. The numbers in parentheses in this outline indicate how many questions on the examination assess some aspect of knowledge in the designated area. The value to you is that this information will help you determine how much time and effort to spend on certain topics. Without using this information as a guide, you may waste valuable time learning information that is not included on the examination. However, we are not suggesting that you deviate from the curriculum established by your state agency or by your teacher. This guide is to help you prepare for the state licensure examination, not to prepare you to work in your practice area. You will need skills that cannot be directly assessed by a written examination.

The simulated examination for bone densitometry equipment operators licensure is located after the ARRT Content Specifications in this section. You should schedule time to complete the entire examination at one sitting. This will give you experience completing an examination of that length and give you some idea of how long it will take you to do so.

The simulated examination consists of 60 questions, as prescribed in the ARRT Content Specifications, and contains the appropriate number of questions from each of the eight content areas: basic concepts (12), equipment operation and QC (9), radiation safety (9), and DXA scanning of the finger (4), heel (os calcis) (4), forearm (6), lumbar spine (8), and proximal femur (8). The questions are further focused to cover content specified in the outline for each content area. You will see that there are more content topics in each outline than there are questions included in the examination. This means that some content will not be assessed with a question, both on the simulated examination and on your actual state licensure examination. That is why it is important for you to review all topics included in each content outline in the ARRT Content Specifications. You cannot rely only on the simulated examination to prepare you for your state licensure examination.

The answers to all simulated examination questions are located after the last question. We have included the correct answer (ANS), as well as the textbook chapter in *Radiography Essentials for Limited Practice* in which the information is located (REF), the designator for the ARRT Content Specifications topic outline item that the question is designed to assess (OBJ), and the topic (TOP) addressed by each question. This information will allow you to easily find and review text material that you have not yet mastered.

Your timeline to prepare for the state licensure examination should be something like the following:

- Participate in the educational program.
- Complete all workbook exercises related to the area of practice. Don't waste time on radiographic procedures chapters outside your licensure area. This activity is especially important if you are not in a formal education program.

- Complete the simulated examination.
- Analyze the results of your examination to identify information you have not yet mastered.
- Review information related to questions you missed on the examination. It may be helpful to repeat relevant workbook exercises.
- Complete the simulated examination again and analyze the results. Review additional information, as needed.
- Successfully complete the state limited scope licensure examination!

ARRT Content Specifications for the Bone Densitometry Equipment Operators Examination

CONTENT SPECIFICATIONS FOR THE BONE DENSITOMETRY EQUIPMENT OPERATORS EXAMINATION

Content Specifications Effective with the January 2003 Examination

The Bone Densitometry Equipment Operator Examination is made available to state licensing agencies to assess the knowledge and cognitive skills required to perform DXA scans of central and peripheral anatomical sites. These content specifications were derived from the ARRT Job Analysis Project for Bone Densitometry. The ARRT administers the examination to state approved candidates under contractual arrangement and provides the results directly to the state. This examination is not associated with any type of certification by the ARRT.

The major sections of the examination are outlined below. Subsequent pages describe in detail the topics covered within each major section.

Section		Number of Questions
A.	Basic Concepts	12
B.	Equipment Operation & QC	9
C.	Radiation Safety	9
D.	DXA Scanning of Finger	4
E.	DXA Scanning of Heel (Os Calcis)	4
F.	DXA Scanning of Forearm	6
G.	DXA Scanning of Lumbar Spine	8
H.	DXA Scanning of Proximal Femur	8
		60*

*An additional 20% of the test may be pilot questions.

A. BASIC CONCEPTS (12)

1. **Osteoporosis**
   a. World Health Organization (WHO) Definition and Diagnostic Criteria
   b. Primary vs. Secondary
   c. Type I (postmenopausal) vs. Type II (senile)
   d. Risk Factors
      1) Controllable (smoking, calcium intake, estrogen, medications)
      2) Uncontrollable (heredity, race, gender, age, medical conditions)

2. **Bone Physiology**
   a. Functions of Bone
      1) structural support & protection
      2) storage of essential minerals
   b. Types of Bone
      1) cortical bone
      2) trabecular bone
   c. Bone Remodeling Cycle
      1) resorption/formation
      2) osteoblasts/osteoclasts
   d. Bone Health
      1) nutrition
      2) exercise

3. **BMD Testing Methods** (anatomical sites scanned; key advantages and disadvantages)
   a. Dual-Energy X-ray Absorptiometry (DXA)
   b. Single X-ray Absorptiometry (SXA)
   c. Quantitative Ultrasound (QUS)
   d. Radiographic Absorptiometry (RA)

4. **Measuring BMD**
   a. Basic Statistical Concepts
      1) mean
      2) standard deviation
      3) coefficient of variation
   b. Reporting Patient Results
      1) BMD formula
      2) Z-score
      3) T-score

B. EQUIPMENT OPERATION & QC (9)

1. **Computer Console**
   a. Major Components
   b. File Management

2. **Fundamentals of X-ray Production**
   a. Properties of X-ray Beam
      1) quality (kVp)
      2) quantity (mA)
      3) duration/time (S)
   b. Filters and Collimators
   c. X-ray Energy Production
      1) single
      2) dual

3. **Types of DXA Systems**
   a. Pencil Beam Systems
   b. Fan Beam Systems
   c. Cone Beam Systems

4. **Quality Control**
   a. Equipment Safety (electrical, pinch points, emergency stop)
   b. Use of Phantoms and/or Calibration
   c. Troubleshooting
      1) shift or drift
      2) pass/fail
   d. Record Maintenance

5. **Determining Quality in BMD**
   a. Precision (definition)
   b. Accuracy (definition)
   c. Factors Affecting Accuracy and Precision
      1) scanner
      2) operator
      3) patient

C. RADIATION SAFETY (9)

1. **Fundamental Principles**
   a. ALARA
   b. Basic Methods of Protection
      1) time
      2) distance
      3) shielding

2. **Biological Effects of Radiation**
   a. Long-Term Effects
      1) cancer
      2) cataracts
      3) life-shortening
   b. Radiosensitive Tissues/Organs

3. **Units of Measurement**
   a. Absorbed Dose
      1) Rad
      2) Gray (Gy, mGy, µGy)
   b. Exposure (dose equivalent)
      1) rem, mrem
      2) Sievert (Sv, mSv, µSv)

4. **Radiation Protection in BD**
   a. General Protection Issues
      1) radiation signs posted
      2) door closed
      3) only patient and operator in room
   b. Occupational Protection
      1) scanner-operator distance
      2) personnel monitoring
      3) exposure records
   c. Patient Protection
      1) comparison levels of radiation
         a. peripheral DXA
         b. central DXA
         c. natural background radiation
         d. airline flight
         e. chest x-ray
      2) Strategies to minimize patient exposure
         a. patient instructions
         b. correct exam performance

D. DXA SCANNING OF FINGER (4)

1. **Anatomy**
   a. Regions of Interest
   b. Bony Landmarks
   c. Radiographic Appearance
   d. Adjacent Structures

2. **Scan Acquisition**
   a. Patient Instructions
   b. Patient Positioning
   c. Evaluating Pre-Set Scan Parameters

3. **Scan Analysis**
   a. BMD
   b. T-score, Z-score

4. **Common Problems**
   a. Nonremovable Artifacts
   b. Fractures or Pathology

E. DXA SCANNING OF HEEL (OS CALCIS) (4)

1. Anatomy
   a. Regions of Interest
   b. Bony Landmarks
   c. Radiographic Appearance
   d. Adjacent Structures

2. Scan Acquisition
   a. Patient Instructions
   b. Patient Positioning
   c. Evaluating Pre-Set Scan Parameters

3. Scan Analysis
   a. BMD
   b. T-score, Z-score

4. Common Problems
   a. Nonremovable Artifacts
   b. Fractures or Pathology

F. DXA SCANNING OF FOREARM (6)

1. Anatomy
   a. Regions of Interest
   b. Bony Landmarks
   c. Radiographic Appearance
   d. Adjacent Structures

2. Scan Acquisition
   a. Patient Instructions
   b. Patient Positioning
   c. Evaluating Pre-Set Scan Parameters

3. Scan Analysis
   a. Accurate ROI Placement
   b. BMC, Area, and BMD
   c. T-score, Z-score

4. Common Problems
   a. Poor Bone Edge Detection
   b. Nonremovable Artifacts
   c. Variant Anatomy
   d. Fractures or Pathology

5. Follow-Up Scans
   a. Unit of Comparison
      1) BMD
      2) T-score
   b. Reproduce Baseline Study

G. DXA SCANNING OF LUMBAR SPINE (8)

1. **Anatomy**
   a. Regions of Interest
   b. Bony Landmarks
   c. Radiographic Appearance
   d. Adjacent Structures

2. **Scan Acquisition**
   a. Patient Instructions
   b. Patient Positioning
   c. Evaluating Pre-Set Scan Parameters

3. **Scan Analysis and Printout**
   a. Accurate ROI Placement
   b. BMC, Area, and BMD
   c. T-score, Z-score

4. **Common Problems**
   a. Poor Bone Edge Detection
   b. Nonremovable Artifacts
   c. Variant Anatomy
   d. Fractures or Pathology

5. **Follow-Up Scans**
   a. Unit of Comparison
      1) BMD
      2) T-score
   b. Reproduce Baseline Study

H. DXA SCANNING OF PROXIMAL FEMUR (8)

1. **Anatomy**
   a. Regions of Interest
   b. Bony Landmarks
   c. Radiographic Appearance
   d. Adjacent Structures

2. **Scan Acquisition**
   a. Patient Instructions
   b. Patient Positioning
   c. Evaluating Pre-Set Scan Parameters

3. **Scan Analysis and Printout**
   a. Accurate ROI Placement
   b. BMC, Area, and BMD
   c. T-score, Z-score

4. **Common Problems**
   a. Poor Bone Edge Detection
   b. Nonremovable Artifacts
   c. Variant Anatomy
   d. Fractures or Pathology

5. **Follow-Up Scans**
   a. Unit of Comparison
      1) BMD
      2) T-score
   b. Reproduce Baseline Study

Simulated Examination for Bone Densitometry Equipment Operators Licensure

Simulated Examination for Bone Densitometry Equipment Operators Licensure

Complete this examination in pencil if you plan to take it more than once. If you are not sure of the answer to a question, skip it and return to it after completing the entire examination.

Multiple Choice

Identify the choice that best completes the statement or answers the question.

_____ 1. According to the World Health Organization (WHO) what bone density level T-score indicates osteoporosis?
    A. +1 to –1
    B. –1 to –2.5
    C. Greater than 2.5
    D. None, there is no correlation

_____ 2. Primary type I osteoporosis is classified as:
    A. premenopausal.
    B. postmenopausal.
    C. senile.
    D. rheumatoid.

_____ 3. Which of the following is an uncontrollable risk factor for osteoporosis?
    A. Gender
    B. Estrogen deficiency
    C. Low calcium intake
    D. Smoking

_____ 4. What are the two basic types of bone?
    A. Cortical and trabecular
    B. Flat and round
    C. Long and short
    D. Simple and complex

_____ 5. Which of the following cells are responsible for building bone?
    A. Osteotytes
    B. Osteolytes
    C. Osteoclasts
    D. Osteoblasts

_____ 6. Bone health requires adequate intake and absorption of what two substances?
    A. Calcium and potassium
    B. Calcium and vitamin D
    C. Potassium and vitamin D
    D. Vitamin D and vitamin E

_____ 7. Which of the following body parts is *not* usually scanned when dual energy x-ray absorptiometry (DXA) scanning is performed?
    A. Lumbar spine
    B. Knee
    C. Proximal femur (hip)
    D. Forearm

_____ 8. Which BMD testing method is considered the gold standard for diagnosis and monitoring of osteoporosis?
    A. Quantitative ultrasound (QUS)
    B. Radiographic absorptiometry (RA)
    C. Single energy x-ray absorptiometry (SXA)
    D. Dual energy x-ray absorptiometry (DXA)

_____ 9. What does BMD stand for, as it relates to osteoporosis testing?
    A. Body mass determination
    B. Bone mineral density
    C. Bone muscle distribution
    D. Biomass density

____ 10. Which of the following is *not* one of the three basic statistical concepts utilized in measuring BMD?
   A. Mean
   B. Median
   C. Standard deviation
   D. Coefficient of variation

____ 11. Which BMD measurement score indicates the number of standard deviations from the average BMD of young, normal, sex-matched individuals with peak bone mass?
   A. T-score
   B. W-score
   C. V-score
   D. Z-score

____ 12. Which BMD measurement score indicates the number of standard deviations from the average BMD for the patient's respective age and sex group?
   A. T-score
   B. W-score
   C. V-score
   D. Z-score

____ 13. Which prime factor of x-ray production, selected by the limited operator, controls the quality or penetrating property?
   A. Milliamperage (mA)
   B. Milliampere-seconds (mAs)
   C. Seconds
   D. Kilovoltage (kVp)

____ 14. Which prime factor of x-ray production, selected by the limited operator, controls the quantity or intensity property?
   A. mA
   B. Seconds
   C. kVp
   D. Filtration

____ 15. For bone densitometry modalities requiring a dual energy x-ray beam, what device is used to create the two photon energy levels?
   A. Collimator
   B. Filter
   C. Grid
   D. Fan

____ 16. DXA bone densitometry requires how many photon energy levels?
   A. One
   B. Two
   C. Three
   D. Four

____ 17. Which of the following is *not* a type of DXA system beam geometry?
   A. Pencil beam
   B. Fan beam
   C. Cone beam
   D. Trough beam

____ 18. Which quantitative performance measure is most important in following a patient's BMD over time?
   A. Stability
   B. Accuracy
   C. Geometry
   D. Precision

____ 19. Scanner quality control (QC) to detect shift or drift is accomplished by imaging what object?
   A. Phantom
   B. Filter
   C. Grid
   D. Patient

____ 20. When, during the day, should daily scanner QC be performed on a normally functioning scanner?
   A. Before the first patient
   B. Between each patient
   C. Between every fifth patient
   D. After the last patient only

____ 21. Which of the following is an operator-controlled factor affecting precision?
   A. Geometric factors on the array scanner
   B. Stability of scanner calibration
   C. Region of interest (ROI) placement
   D. Patient anatomic variations

____ 22. The acronym *ALARA* stands for what radiation protection principle?
   A. As Long As Reasonably Allowed
   B. As Long As Realistically Achievable
   C. As Low As Reasonably Achievable
   D. As Low As Realistically Allowed

____ 23. What are the three basic factors that can be manipulated to minimize radiation exposure?
   A. Time, distance, shielding
   B. Filtration, time, shielding
   C. Distance, collimation, filtration
   D. Time, collimation, filtration

____ 24. What is the unit of absorbed dose, in addition to the rad?
   A. rem
   B. sievert
   C. gray
   D. roentgen

____ 25. What is the unit of effective dose (equivalent), in addition to the rem?
  A. rad
  B. sievert
  C. gray
  D. roentgen

____ 26. Which of the following is a general radiation safety guideline for DXA scanning?
  A. A lead shield should be provided to each patient.
  B. The operator computer console should be in contact with the scanning table.
  C. A radiation sign should be posted outside the scanning room.
  D. Questionable scans should never be repeated.

____ 27. Which of the following is an operator radiation safety guideline for DXA scanning?
  A. A lead shield should be worn by the operator.
  B. The operator computer console should be in contact with the scanning table.
  C. The operator should leave the room during scan data acquisition.
  D. The operator should wear a dosimetry device at the collar.

____ 28. Which of the following is the highest radiation source?
  A. A PA chest radiograph
  B. A roundtrip airline flight
  C. Daily natural background radiation
  D. DXA scan of the forearm

____ 29. Which of the following is the lowest radiation source?
  A. A PA chest radiograph
  B. A roundtrip airline flight
  C. Daily natural background radiation
  D. DXA scan of the forearm

____ 30. Which of the following is a potential long-term effect of radiation exposure?
  A. Cancer
  B. Skin reddening
  C. Significant, rapid hair loss
  D. Sudden intestinal bleeding

____ 31. What is the ROI used for DXA scanning of the finger?
  A. Proximal phalanx
  B. Middle phalanx
  C. Distal phalanx
  D. Entire digit

____ 32. How is the hand positioned for DXA scanning of the finger?
  A. Palm up
  B. Palm down
  C. Resting on medial side
  D. Resting on lateral side

____ 33. Which of the following conditions of the patient's finger will adversely effect the results of a DXA scan?
  1. Fracture or arthritis in the scanner field of view
  2. Ring located in the scanner field of view
  3. Nonmetallic fingernail polish on the finger to be scanned
  A. 1 and 2 only
  B. 1 and 3 only
  C. 2 and 3 only
  D. 1, 2, and 3

____ 34. Which hand should be used for DXA scanning of the finger?
  A. Dominant hand
  B. Nondominant hand
  C. Always the right hand
  D. Always the left hand

____ 35. Which type of DXA scanning is performed on the heel (calcaneus or os calcis)?
  A. Central
  B. Peripheral

____ 36. DXA scanning is commonly performed on which heel(s)?
  A. Left
  B. Right
  C. Both

____ 37. Which of the following body parts can be scanned with cone-beam DXA technology?
  A. Heel (calcaneus or os calcis)
  B. Lumbar spine
  C. Proximal femur
  D. Forearm

____ 38. Which of the following statements about heel DXA is correct?
  A. Heel DXA is superior to hip DXA for prediction of overall risk of fragility fracture.
  B. Heel DXA is approximately equal to hip DXA for prediction of overall risk of fragility fracture.
  C. Heel DXA is an accepted method for following skeletal response to therapy.
  D. Heel DXA is always performed on the left heel.

____ 39. What is the preferred ROI for a forearm DXA scan?
  A. Proximal third
  B. Middle third
  C. Distal third
  D. Distal half

____ 40. What is the recommended procedure for determining the ROI for a forearm DXA scan?
  A. The ROI consists of the distal one-third of the measured distance from the ulnar styloid to the olecranon process.
  B. The ROI consists of the proximal one-third of the measured distance from the ulnar styloid to the olecranon process.
  C. The ROI consists of the middle one-third of the measured distance from the ulnar styloid to the olecranon process.
  D. The ROI consists of the distal one-third of the measured distance from the radial styloid to the olecranon process.

____ 41. What is a common error that creates a problem in placement of the one-third region for a forearm DXA scan?
  A. Scan is too long in the distal direction.
  B. Scan is too short in the distal direction.
  C. Scan is too long in the proximal direction.
  D. Scan is too short in the proximal direction.

____ 42. What is an important problem associated with the ultradistal ROI for forearm DXA scanning?
  A. Poor ROI replication on follow-up scans
  B. Motion
  C. Poor bone edge detection
  D. Artifact formation

____ 43. What condition makes a forearm unsuitable for DXA scanning?
  A. Excessive muscularity
  B. Excessive length
  C. History of localized skin infection
  D. History of fracture

____ 44. Why should the baseline measurement be recorded for a forearm DXA scan?
  A. To ensure proper ROI placement on follow-up scans
  B. To provide diagnostic data for follow-up scans
  C. To prevent malpractice lawsuits
  D. No record is needed

____ 45. What are the ROIs for a lumbar spine DXA scan?
  A. T12 through L3
  B. L1 through L4
  C. L1 through L5
  D. L2 through L5

____ 46. Which of the following is an excellent external landmark for consistent placement of the intervertebral markers at baseline and follow-up lumbar spine DXA scanning?
  A. L4 spinous process
  B. Iliac crest
  C. Xiphoid process
  D. Greater trochanter

____ 47. Which of the following patient instructions will help ensure an artifact-free lumbar spine DXA scan?
  A. Hold your breath.
  B. Remove your clothing and change into an examination gown.
  C. Remove any dentures or partial plates.
  D. Place your hands and arms on the table pad.

____ 48. What positioning aid is typically used during lumbar spine DXA scanning?
  A. Positioning leg block
  B. Positioning spine block
  C. Gonad shielding
  D. Measurement calipers

____ 49. Which vertebra has an H or X appearance on a lumbar spine DXA scan and aids in proper labeling of vertebral levels?
  A. L2
  B. L3
  C. L4
  D. L5

____ 50. Lumbar spine DXA scans are most appropriate for predicting vertebral fracture risk in patients younger than what age?
  A. 55
  B. 60
  C. 65
  D. 70

____ 51. Which of the following variant anatomy can result in falsely elevated BMD on lumbar spine DXA scans?
  A. Scoliosis
  B. Kyphosis
  C. Lordosis
  D. Spina bifida

____ 52. Which of the following is a unit of comparison for serial lumbar spine DXA scans?
  A. Osteoporosis
  B. X-score
  C. BMD
  D. ROI

_____ 53. Where is the ROI located for DXA scanning of the proximal femur?
   A. Femoral neck
   B. Femoral head
   C. Greater trochanter
   D. Lesser trochanter

_____ 54. Which of the following part positioning maneuvers can relieve overlap of the ischium and femoral neck?
   A. Leg adduction
   B. Leg abduction
   C. Leg external rotation
   D. Knee flexion

_____ 55. Which anatomic relationship problem results in a falsely elevated femoral neck BMD?
   A. Overlap of the femoral head and neck
   B. Overlap of the greater and lesser trochanters
   C. Overlap of the femoral head and pubis
   D. Overlap of the femoral neck and ischium

_____ 56. Which of the following patient instructions will help ensure an artifact-free DXA scan of the proximal femur?
   A. Hold your breath.
   B. Remove your clothing and change into an examination gown.
   C. Remove any dentures or partial plates.
   D. Place your hands and arms on the table pad.

_____ 57. Which of the following external landmarks are used to properly place the laser centering light for a DXA scan of the proximal femur?
   A. Iliac crest and pubic symphysis
   B. Pubic symphysis and greater trochanter
   C. Greater trochanter and lesser trochanter
   D. Lesser trochanter and iliac crest

_____ 58. Proper comparison of hip BMD over time requires that the angle of the femoral neck box ROI to be the same in serial scans. To accomplish this, what two femoral structures must appear identical on follow-up DXA scans of the proximal femur?
   A. Lesser trochanter and femoral body (shaft)
   B. Ischium and femoral head
   C. Femoral head and greater trochanter
   D. Ischium and pubic symphysis

_____ 59. If osteoarthritis of the hip is present, what adjustments in scan protocol should be made during a DXA scan of the proximal femur?
   A. Always scan the left hip.
   B. Always scan the nondominant hip.
   C. Scan the less affected hip.
   D. Scan the more affected hip.

_____ 60. What are the two ROIs for a DXA scan of the proximal femur?
   A. Femoral neck and total hip
   B. Femoral neck and total femur
   C. Femoral head and greater trochanter
   D. Greater trochanter and ischium

Simulated Examination for Bone Densitometry Equipment Operators Licensure

Answer Section

Multiple Choice:

1. **ANS: C**	REF: Ch. 28	OBJ: exam spec A.a.1	TOP: osteoporosis
2. **ANS: B**	REF: Ch. 28	OBJ: exam spec A.1.c	TOP: osteoporosis
3. **ANS: A**	REF: Ch. 28	OBJ: exam spec A.1.d	TOP: osteoporosis
4. **ANS: A**	REF: Ch. 28	OBJ: exam spec A.2.b	TOP: bone physiology
5. **ANS: D**	REF: Ch. 28	OBJ: exam spec A.2.c	TOP: bone physiology
6. **ANS: B**	REF: Ch. 28	OBJ: exam spec A.2.d.1	TOP: bone physiology
7. **ANS: B**	REF: Ch. 28	OBJ: exam spec A.3.a	TOP: BMD testing methods
8. **ANS: D**	REF: Ch. 28	OBJ: exam spec A.3	TOP: BMD testing methods
9. **ANS: B**	REF: Ch. 28	OBJ: exam spec A.3	TOP: BMD testing methods
10. **ANS: B**	REF: Ch. 28	OBJ: exam spec A.4.a	TOP: measuring BMD
11. **ANS: A**	REF: Ch. 28	OBJ: exam spec A.4.b.2	TOP: measuring BMD
12. **ANS: D**	REF: Ch. 28	OBJ: exam spec A.4.b.3	TOP: measuring BMD
13. **ANS: D**	REF: Ch. 28	OBJ: exam spec B.2.a.1	TOP: fundamentals of x-ray production
14. **ANS: A**	REF: Ch. 28	OBJ: exam spec B.2.a.2	TOP: fundamentals of x-ray production
15. **ANS: B**	REF: Ch. 28	OBJ: exam spec B.2.b	TOP: fundamentals of x-ray production
16. **ANS: B**	REF: Ch. 28	OBJ: exam spec B.2.c.2	TOP: fundamentals of x-ray production
17. **ANS: D**	REF: Ch. 28	OBJ: exam spec B.3	TOP: DXA system types

18. **ANS: D**	REF: Ch. 28	OBJ: exam spec B.5.a	TOP: determining quality in BMD
19. **ANS: A**	REF: Ch. 28	OBJ: exam spec B.4.b	TOP: determining quality in BMD
20. **ANS: A**	REF: Ch. 28	OBJ: exam spec B.4	TOP: quality control
21. **ANS: C**	REF: Ch. 28	OBJ: exam spec B.5.c.2	TOP: determining quality in BMD
22. **ANS: C**	REF: Ch. 28	OBJ: exam spec C.1.a	TOP: radiation safety principles
23. **ANS: A**	REF: Ch. 28	OBJ: exam spec C.1.b	TOP: radiation safety principles
24. **ANS: C**	REF: Ch. 28	OBJ: exam spec C.3.a	TOP: radiation units
25. **ANS: B**	REF: Ch. 28	OBJ: exam spec C.3.b	TOP: radiation units
26. **ANS: C**	REF: Ch. 28	OBJ: exam spec C.4.a	TOP: radiation protection in BD
27. **ANS: D**	REF: Ch. 28	OBJ: exam spec C.4.b	TOP: radiation protection in BD
28. **ANS: B**	REF: Ch. 28	OBJ: exam spec C.4.c	TOP: radiation protection in BD
29. **ANS: D**	REF: Ch. 28	OBJ: exam spec C.4.c	TOP: radiation protection in BD
30. **ANS: A**	REF: Ch. 13	OBJ: exam spec C.2.a	TOP: biological effects of radiation
31. **ANS: B**	REF: Ch. 28	OBJ: exam spec D.1.a	TOP: finger DXA ROI
32. **ANS: B**	REF: Ch. 28	OBJ: exam spec D.2.b	TOP: finger DXA positioning
33. **ANS: A**	REF: Ch. 28	OBJ: exam spec D.4	TOP: finger DXA common problems
34. **ANS: B**	REF: Ch. 28	OBJ: exam spec D.2.b	TOP: finger DXA positioning
35. **ANS: B**	REF: Ch. 28	OBJ: exam spec E.2	TOP: heel DXA scan acquisition
36. **ANS: B**	REF: Ch. 28	OBJ: exam spec E.2.b	TOP: heel DXA positioning
37. **ANS: A**	REF: Ch. 28	OBJ: exam spec E.2	TOP: heel DXA acquisition
38. **ANS: B**	REF: Ch. 28	OBJ: exam spec E.3.a	TOP: heel DXA scan analysis
39. **ANS: C**	REF: Ch. 28	OBJ: exam spec F.1.a	TOP: forearm DXA anatomy
40. **ANS: A**	REF: Ch. 28	OBJ: exam spec F.2.b	TOP: forearm DXA scan acquisition
41. **ANS: D**	REF: Ch. 28	OBJ: exam spec F.3.a	TOP: forearm DXA scan analysis
42. **ANS: C**	REF: Ch. 28	OBJ: exam spec F.4.a	TOP: forearm DXA common problems
43. **ANS: D**	REF: Ch. 28	OBJ: exam spec F.4.d	TOP: forearm DXA common problems
44. **ANS: A**	REF: Ch. 28	OBJ: exam spec F.5.b	TOP: forearm DXA follow-up scans
45. **ANS: B**	REF: Ch. 28	OBJ: exam spec G.1.a	TOP: lumber spine DXA anatomy
46. **ANS: B**	REF: Ch. 28	OBJ: exam spec G.1.b	TOP: lumbar spine DXA anatomy
47. **ANS: B**	REF: Ch. 28	OBJ: exam spec G.2.a	TOP: lumbar spine DXA scan acquisition
48. **ANS: A**	REF: Ch. 28	OBJ: exam spec G.2.b	TOP: lumbar spine DXA scan acquisition
49. **ANS: C**	REF: Ch. 28	OBJ: exam spec G.3.a, G.1.c	TOP: lumbar spine DXA scan analysis and anatomy
50. **ANS: C**	REF: Ch. 28	OBJ: exam spec G.3.b	TOP: lumbar spine DXA scan analysis
51. **ANS: A**	REF: Ch. 28	OBJ: exam spec G.4.c	TOP: lumbar spine DXA scan common problems
52. **ANS: C**	REF: Ch. 28	OBJ: exam spec G.5.a.1	TOP: lumbar spine DXA scan follow-up
53. **ANS: A**	REF: Ch. 28	OBJ: exam spec H.1.a	TOP: proximal femur DXA scan anatomy
54. **ANS: B**	REF: Ch. 28	OBJ: exam spec H.2.b	TOP: proximal femur DXA scan acquisition
55. **ANS: D**	REF: Ch. 28	OBJ: exam spec H.3.b, H.1.d	TOP: proximal femur DXA scan analysis and anatomy
56. **ANS: B**	REF: Ch. 28	OBJ: exam spec H.2.a	TOP: proximal femur DXA scan acquisition
57. **ANS: B**	REF: Ch. 28	OBJ: exam spec H.1.b	TOP: proximal femur DXA scan anatomy
58. **ANS: A**	REF: Ch. 28	OBJ: exam spec H.5.b, H.3.a, H.1.c	TOP: proximal femur DXA scan follow-up, analysis, and anatomy
59. **ANS: C**	REF: Ch. 28	OBJ: exam spec H.4.d	TOP: proximal femur DXA scan common problems
60. **ANS: A**	REF: Ch. 28	OBJ: exam spec H.1.a, H.3.a	TOP: proximal femur DXA scan analysis and anatomy

Answers to Section I

Chapter 1

Exercise 1

1. D

2. A

3. C

4. True

5. A

6. B

7. D

8. D

9. A

10. C

11. B

12. B

13. B

14. False

15. True

Exercise 2

1. X-rays were discovered in 1895 by Wilhelm Conrad Roentgen at the University of Wurzburg in Germany.

2. The purpose of ARRT is to establish qualifications, administer examinations, and provide certification for professional radiologic technologists. This organization also provides limited scope examinations to states that provide certifications for limited scope x-ray machine operators. In addition, ARRT publishes the Code of Ethics and Rules of Ethics for professional radiographers, which are the existing standard of practice for radiography. While these standards do not apply directly to limited operators, they should be seen as the prevailing standards for appropriate conduct by limited operators and radiographers.

3. Licenses or permits may be suspended or revoked. Fines and/or imprisonment may be levied against the limited operator and/or the employer.

4. The professional credential is RT(R), and it stands for "registered technologist (radiography)."

5. Reciprocity is the recognition of credentials acquired in one state by other states. Reciprocity facilitates the ability of limited radiographers to qualify to practice when moving from state to state.

6. Front office activities: greeting patients, making appointments, handling payments, handling insurance and billing, and filing records

   Back office activities: consultation, examination, treatment, laboratory testing, and radiography

7. Explain radiographic procedures to patients.

   Measure parts to be radiographed.

   Determine exposure factors and set the control panel.

   Position the patient correctly for the examination.

   Position the x-ray tube correctly for the examination.

   Position the film correctly for the examination.

   Process the radiographic film.

   Evaluate the processed film for quality.

   Prepare the films for reading by the physician.

Exercise 3

1. D

2. G

3. H

4. E

5. C

6. F

7. A

8. B

Exercise 4

1. F
2. B
3. A
4. E
5. C
6. D
7. H
8. G

Chapter 2

Exercise 1

1. C
2. D
3. C
4. B
5. D
6. A
7. B
8. A
9. C
10. A
11. D

Exercise 2

1. Turn on the collimator light. The crosshairs in the center of the illuminated radiation field indicates the location of the central ray.

2. Between the patient and the film, on the side of the patient opposite that of the x-ray tube.

3. *Attenuation* is the term used to refer to absorption of the x-ray beam. Attenuation results in the production of scattered radiation.

4. The control console, also called the *control panel*.

5. Release the appropriate lock(s).

6. On the underside of the x-ray tube housing

7. By reading the scale on the face of the collimator

8. Before making an exposure, be certain of the following:
   The x-ray room door is closed.
   No nonessential persons are in the x-ray room.
   All persons in the control booth are completely behind the lead barrier.
   No cassettes are in the room except the one in use.

9. Immediately. X-rays travel at the speed of light and do not linger in the room. They are present only during an exposure.

10. *Primary radiation* is defined as the x-ray beam that leaves the tube and is unattenuated, except by air. Its direction and location are predictable and controllable. *Remnant radiation* is what remains of the primary beam after it has been attenuated by matter. Since the pattern of densities in the matter results in differential absorption of the radiation, this pattern will be inherent in the remnant radiation. The pattern of the remnant radiation creates the film image.

11. The 8 × 10 inch and 10 × 12 inch are still manufactured in English sizes.

12. The patient is placed on the x-ray table and the table is tilted so the head is lower than the feet. The angle is typically at least 15 degrees.

13. The latent image is the unseen image that is on the film after exposure.

Exercise 3

1. C
2. F
3. A
4. G
5. B
6. D
7. E

Chapter 3

Exercise 1

1. C

2. F

3. B

4. G

5. D

6. E

7. A

Exercise 2

1. Denominator

2. Numerator

3. Whole number, fraction

4. Numerator of the fraction, denominator of the fraction

5. A. 8
   B. 30
   C. 60
   D. 75
   E. 70

6. A. 2/5
   B. 1/4
   C. 1/3
   D. 1/3
   E. 1/3
   F. 3/5
   G. 3/4

7. Whole numbers

8. Tenths (10ths); hundredths (100ths); thousandths (1000ths)

9. True

10. False

11. A. $\begin{array}{r} 21.70 \\ +5.39 \\ \hline 27.09 \end{array}$

B. $\begin{array}{r} 33.06 \\ +30.20 \\ \hline 63.26 \end{array}$

C. $\begin{array}{r} 14.911 \\ +208.700 \\ \hline 223.611 \end{array}$

D. $\begin{array}{r} 29.844 \\ 3.300 \\ +27.600 \\ \hline 60.744 \end{array}$

E. $\begin{array}{r} 285.200 \\ 46.910 \\ +11.402 \\ \hline 343.512 \end{array}$

12. A. $\begin{array}{r} 335.65 \\ -46.23 \\ \hline 289.42 \end{array}$

B. $\begin{array}{r} 456.33 \\ -3.87 \\ \hline 452.46 \end{array}$

C. $\begin{array}{r} 39.800 \\ -6.323 \\ \hline 33.477 \end{array}$

D. $\begin{array}{r} 21.00 \\ -7.51 \\ \hline 13.49 \end{array}$

E. $\begin{array}{r} 19.042 \\ -4.120 \\ \hline 14.922 \end{array}$

13. Count the total number of decimal places in the numbers that are being multiplied. This is the number of decimal places that should be in the product before any zeros are dropped. For example, when a number with one decimal place is multiplied by a number with two decimal places, the product should have three decimal places.

14. A. $\begin{array}{r} 29.5 \\ \times 5 \\ \hline 147.5 \end{array}$

B. $\begin{array}{r} 17.6 \\ \times 40 \\ \hline 704.0 \end{array}$

C.   341.225
      ×48.33
      1023675
      1023675
      2729800
      1364900
      16491.40425

D.   0.2213
      ×82.7
      15491
      4426
      17704
      18.30151

E.   83.22
      ×906.1
      8322
      49932
      748980
      75405.642

15. A.   6.9
          5)34.5

B.   72.035
      10)720.350
          70
          20
          20
          03
          0
          35
          30
          50
          50
          0

C.   11.6
      2.5)29.00
          25
          40
          25
          150
          150
          0

D.   70.2
      4.05)284.310
          2835
          81
          0
          810
          810
          0

E.   98
      6.22)609.56
          5598
          4976
          4976
          0

16. Numerator; denominator

17. A. 0.125

    B. 0.375

    C. 0.0166 …

    D. 0.1333 …

    E. 1.25

18. Right to left

19. 5; 4

20. A. 1.67

    B. 0.7414

    C. 0.25

    D. 3.255

    E. 10.44

21. A. $^1/_4$ = 0.25 $^1/_{20}$ = 0.05 $^2/_3$ = 0.667
       0.25 + 0.05 + 0.667 = 0.967
    B. $^3/_{10}$ = 0.3 $^1/_5$ = 0.2 $^1/_2$ = 0.5
       0.3 + 0.2 + 0.5 = 1.0
    C. $^3/_4$ = 0.753/8 = 0.375
       0.75 - 0.375 = 0.375
    D. $^2/_{15}$ = 1.333   1.333 × 200 = 266.6
    E. $^3/_5$ = 0.6 $^1/_2$ = 0.5   0.6 ÷ 0.5 = 1.2

22. False

23. True

24. A. 0.2

    B. 0.713

    C. 0.85

    D. 0.69

    E. 1.72

    F. 8

25. A. 33%

    B. 40%

    C. 6%

    D. 189%

    E. 230%

    F. 600%

26. A. 73% + 27% = 100%

    B. 50% + 25% = 75%

    C. 30% - 3% = 27%

    D. 20% × 60% = 0.2 × 0.6 = 0.12 or 12%

    E. 79% × 30% = 0.79 × 0.3 = 0.237 or 23.7%

    F. 25% ÷ 10% = 0.25 ÷ 0.1 = 2.5 or 250%

    G. 48% ÷ 2% = 0.48 ÷ 0.02 = 24 or 2400%

27. A. 30% = 0.3   0.3 × 27 = 8.1

    B. 95% = 0.95   0.95 × 320 = 304

    C. 50% = 0.5   0.5 × 31 = 15.5

    D. 170% = 1.7   1.7 × 60 = 102

    E. 200% = 2   2 × 20 = 40

28. A. 11 ÷ 64 = 0.1718 = 17.2%

    B. 71 ÷ 90 = 0.7888 ... = 78.9%

    C. 50 ÷ 300 = 0.1666 ... = 16.7%

    D. 40 ÷ 200 = 0.2 = 20%

    E. 70 ÷ 35 = 2.0 = 200%

29. A. 100% + 15% = 115% = 1.15
       1.15 × 75 = 86.25

    B. 100% + 100% = 200% = 2
       2 × 30 = 60

    C. 100% + 20% = 120% = 1.2
       1.2 × 12 = 14.4

    D. 100% - 10% = 90% = 0.9
       0.9 × 85 = 76.5

    E. 100% - 12% = 88% = 0.88
       0.88 × 50 = 44

30. Equation

31. True

32. Divided

33. True

34. Ratio

35. Proportion

36. A. $2x + 9 - 9 = 11 + 3 - 9$
       $2x = 5$
       $2x \div 2 = 5 \div 2$
       $x = 2.5$

    B. $^{16}/x \times x = (12 - 4) \times x 16 = 8x$
       $16 \div 8 = 8x \div 8$
       $2 = x$

    C. $x - 61 + 61 = 12 + 61$
       $x = 73$

    D. $45 + 15 = 4x - 15 + 15$
       $60 = 4x$
       $60 \div 4 = 4x \div 4$
       $15 = x$

    E. $3x \times 3 = 9/3 \times 3$ _
       $9x = 9$
       $9x \div 9 = 9 \div 9$
       $x = 1$

    F. $64 \div 8 = 8x \div 8$
       $8 = x$

    G. $10x = 2 \times 25$
       $10x = 50$
       $10x \div 10 = 50 \div 10$
       $x = 5$

    H. $48x = 3 \times 12$
       $48x = 36$
       $48x \div 48 = 36 \div 48$
       $x = 0.75$

    I. $72x = 8 \times 80$
       $72x = 640$
       $72x \div 72 = 640 \div 72$
       $x = 8.889$

J. $4x = 60$
$4x \div 4 = 60 \div 4$
$x = 15$

37. 4^3

38. 5^5

39. A. $3^2 = 3 \times 3 = 9$

B. $3^3 = 3 \times 3 \times 3 = 27$

C. $2^4 = 2 \times 2 \times 2 \times 2 = 16$

D. $9^2 = 9 \times 9 = 81$

E. $40^2 = 40 \times 40 = 1600$

40. A. 3

B. 4

C. 5

D. 9

E. 12

41. 1. C

2. H

3. F

4. D

5. B

6. E

7. G

8. A

42. A. 3

B. 12

C. 16

D. 2000

E. 16

43. A. 100

B. 1000

C. 1000

D. 0.001

44. A. 70,000 V

B. 500 cm

C. 0.03 L

D. 0.1 kg

E. 0.002 g

45. A. 18 in $\div$ 12 = 1.5 ft   1.5 ft $\div$ 3 ft = 0.5 yd

B. 2 qt $\times$ 2 = 4 pt   4 pt $\times$ 16 = 48 oz

C. 68 in $\div$ 12 = 5.67 ft

D. 20 qt $\div$ 4 = 5 gal

E. 3.5 lb $\times$ 16 = 56 oz

46. A. 5 fl oz $\times$ 30 = 150 ml

B. 100 lb $\times$ 0.45 = 45 kg

C. 14 in $\times$ 2.54 = 35.36 cm
35.36 $\div$ 1000 = 0.0354 m

D. 50 mm $\div$ 10 = 5 cm
5 cm $\times$ 0.39 = 1.95 in

E. 100 g $\times$ 0.0022 = 0.22 lb
0.22 $\times$ 16 = 3.52 oz

47. A. $\frac{1}{60}$ sec = 0.0167 sec
0.0167 $\times$ 1000 = 16.7 msec

B. 260 sec $\div$ 60 = 4.3333 min
4.3333 min $\div$ 60 = 0.0722 hr

C. 2.4 days $\times$ 24 hr/day = 57.6 hr

D. 75 - 32 = 4343 $\div$ 1.8 = 23.89° C

E. 25° $\times$ 1.8 = 4545 + 32 = 77° F

48. The total quantity of the exposure

49. mA $\times$ Time (sec) = mAs

50. mAs ÷ mA = Time (sec)

51. A. 200 mA × 0.05 sec = 10 mAs

    B. 300 mA × 0.25 sec = 75 mAs

    C. 100 mA × 0.7 sec = 70 mAs

    D. 500 mA × $\frac{1}{20}$ sec = 25 mAs

    E. 50 mA × 0.3 sec = 15 mAs

    F. 150 mA × 1.25 sec = 187.5 mAs

    G. 400 mA × 0.002 sec = 0.8 mAs

52. A. 10 mAs ÷ 50 mA = 0.2 sec (or $\frac{1}{5}$ sec)

    B. 40 mAs ÷ 200 mA = 0.2 sec (or $\frac{1}{5}$ sec)

    C. 6 mAs ÷ 300 mA = 0.02 sec

    D. 2 mAs ÷ 100 mA = 0.02 sec

    E. 75 mAs ÷ 400 mA = 0.188 sec

53. $mAs_1/mAs_2 = SID_1^2/SID_2^2$

54. A. 25% or $\frac{1}{4}$ of the original intensity

    B. 225% or $2\frac{1}{4}$ times the original intensity

    C. 36 mAs

    D. 40.83 mAs

    E. 38.88 mAs

55. 2; 3

56. 30%; 20%

57. A. 84 kVp

    B. 78 kVp

    C. 16 mAs

    D. 84.5 mAs

    E. 19.5 mAs

58. Decreased

59. Divide

60. A. 40 mAs, 81 kVp

    B. 60 mAs, 90 kVp

    C. 10 mAs, 69 kVp

    D. 50 mAs, 85 kVp

    E. 15 mAs, 81 kVp

61. Inversely

62. A. 48 mAs

    B. 16 mAs

    C. 64 mAs

    D. 83.33 mAs

    E. 5 mAs

63. Dose/Strength = Volume

64. A. 4 tablets

    B. 3 ml

    C. 4 ml

    D. 2 tablets

    E. 2000 mg (2 g)

65. Body weight = 40 lb × 0.45 = 18 kg body weight
    2 mg/kg × 18 kg = 36 mg prescribed dose
    36 mg ÷ 4 mg/ml = 9 ml volume to administer

Chapter 4

Exercise 1

1. A

2. C

3. B

4. C

5. B

6. C

7. D

8. A

9. C

10. B

11. D

12. A

13. A

14. D

15. D

16. C

17. D

18. False

19. True

20. True

Exercise 2

1. Energy can be neither created nor destroyed, but it can change form.

2. K shell.

3. Ultraviolet rays
   Visible light
   Infrared rays
   Microwaves
   Radar waves
   Television waves
   Radio waves

4. The shorter the wavelength, the more penetrating the beam.

5. *Ionization* is the creation of one or more charged particles that occurs when an electron is added to or subtracted from a neutral atom. The ionizing ability of electromagnetic radiation is determined by wavelength. Wavelengths shorter than 1 nm have sufficient energy to remove an electron from its orbit.

6. Have no mass
   Are highly penetrating and invisible
   Are electrically neutral
   Are polyenergetic and heterogeneous
   Travel in straight lines at the speed of light

Can ionize matter
Cause fluorescence in certain crystals
Cannot be focused with a lens
Affect photographic film
Produce biologic changes in tissues
Produce secondary and scatter radiation

7. The velocity of x-rays is approximately 186,000 miles/sec (3×10^{10} cm/sec). All electromagnetic energy has the same velocity.

8. Current: amperes (A)
   Potential difference: volts (V)
   Electric resistance: ohms (Ω)

9. An ammeter measures the rate of current flow in units of amperes (A).
   A voltmeter measures electric potential in units of volts (V).
   An ammeter is connected in the circuit in series. A voltmeter is connected in parallel.

10. Electric cycle = $\frac{1}{60}$ sec
    Electric impulse = $\frac{1}{120}$ sec

11. The process by which an electric current in one circuit influences a current to flow in a second circuit. Induction occurs because of movement of the magnetic field surrounding the wire in the first circuit with respect to the coils of wire in the second circuit. No other connection exists between the two circuits.

12. To change voltage.

Exercise 3

1. G

2. I

3. F

4. E

5. C

6. H

7. B

8. D

9. J

10. A

Chapter 5

Exercise 1

1. B

2. A

3. A

4. D

5. B

6. D

7. C

8. C

9. A

10. B

11. B

12. B

13. D

14. D

15. D

16. C

17. B

18. D

19. A

20. C

Exercise 2

1. Tungsten, chemical symbol W, is a metal element; it is a large atom with 74 electrons in orbit around its nucleus. It can be readily formed into wire (as for the filament) or a smooth, hard surface (as in the target). It is an excellent target material because it has a high melting point, which enables it to withstand the heat generated at the target. It produces x-ray photons from characteristic and Bremsstrahlung interactions that are a useful part of the primary x-ray beam. Tungsten is a good filament material because it has a high atomic number, so there are many electrons available in its orbits to form the space charge, the source of electrons for x-ray production.

2. *Thermionic emission* refers to the process that causes charged particles to be given off when heat is applied. Application of heat to the filament of the x-ray tube causes negatively charged particles (electrons) to be given off by the tungsten filament material, which supplies a source of free electrons for x-ray production.

3. *Heterogeneous*, as applied to an x-ray beam, means that the x-ray beam contains a wide range of wavelengths. Bremsstrahlung interactions in the anode produce a heterogeneous x-ray beam. Characteristic interactions in the anode always produce the same wavelength.

4. A dual-focus tube has two filaments and two focal spots. A single-focus tube has only one of each.

5. Target angulation of at least 12 degrees is necessary in a general-purpose tube to create a primary x-ray beam that is large enough to cover a standard 35×43 cm IR at a 40-inch SID, which is one of the standard distances for radiography work.

6. Increased kVp results in an x-ray beam with greater energy and greater penetrating power. A kVp increase will cause a decrease (shortening) of the shortest wavelengths in the x-ray beam and therefore a shorter average wavelength in the beam.

7. An increase in mA might be desirable to increase the quantity of the exposure or to permit a shorter exposure time. Higher mA increases tube load and anode heat. Consistent use of the highest mA settings causes the tube to deteriorate more rapidly.

8. 100 mA $\times$ 0.25 sec = 25 mAs. Other possible combinations of mA and time that will produce 25 mAs include 50 mA and 0.50 sec; 200 mA and 0.125 sec; 500 mA and 0.05 sec.

9. 0.5 mm inherent + 1.25 mm additional = 1.75 mm present. The total required is 2.5 mm. Therefore 0.75 mm Al equivalent filtration must be added (2.5 - 1.75).

10. 3400 rpm is the standard anode rotation speed.

11. None. Characteristic radiation can only be produced above 70 kVp.

12. 45%

Exercise 3

Fig. 5-1
1. Tungsten target
2. Heated tungsten filament
3. Pyrex glass envelope
4. Cathode
5. Anode

Fig. 5-2
1. Electron stream size
2. Actual focal spot size
3. Effective focal spot size

Exercise 4

1. 20
2. 5
3. 75
4. 75
5. 50
6. 400
7. 200
8. 100
9. 1
10. ½
11. 2
12. ¾

Chapter 6

Exercise 1

1. A
2. A
3. C
4. C
5. A
6. D

7. B
8. D
9. C
10. C
11. D
12. A
13. B
14. D
15. D
16. B
17. False
18. False
19. True
20. True

Exercise 2

1. Major kVp selector
2. Minor kVp selector
3. mA selector
4. Focal spot selector
5. Anode
6. Cathode

Exercise 3

A. 2
B. 3
C. 1
D. 2
E. 3
F. 2

G. 1

H. 2

I. 1

J. 3

K. 1

L. 1

Exercise 4

1. Fluctuations in line voltage are caused by changes in the power demand in the neighborhood or in the building. If the control console has automatic monitoring and adjustment for line voltage variations, the radiographer does not need to do anything. Older control panels that have a line meter and a line compensation adjustment require the radiographer to check the line meter and make appropriate adjustments in compensation before setting the control for an exposure.

2. The primary purpose of the autotransformer is to serve as the kilovoltage selector. The autotransformer also functions as the line voltage compensator and provides power to other parts of the circuit.

3. The mA selector on the control panel represents a rheostat in the filament circuit. The x-ray circuit is located on the secondary side of the high-voltage transformer.

4. Devices used to provide rectification are called *diodes*. Four are needed to provide full-wave rectification.

5. High-frequency generators produce a more efficient and constant voltage.
   More constant voltage permits shorter exposure times and reduces patient dose.

6. Activate and hold rotor switch.
   On signal, activate and hold exposure switch.
   Observe exposure indicator to validate exposure and to determine when it is complete.
   Release rotor and exposure switches.

7. The anode begins to rotate.
   Full heat is applied to the filament.

8. The copper mass incorporated in the anode conducts heat from the target.

The rotating anode spreads heat over a greater area.
The structural layers of the rotating anode are designed to handle heat effectively.
Oil in the tube housing dissipates heat from the glass envelope.

9. From the points where the 80-kVp line intersects each mA curve, draw a vertical line to the bottom of the graph and read the exposure time. Multiply each mA value by the time associated with it to determine the mAs possible at that mA setting and 80 kVp. The greatest mAs available at 80 kVp is 800 mAs, obtained by using 100 mA and 8 sec.

10. $HU = mA \times sec \times kVp$
    $300 \times 1 \times 90 = 27{,}000 \ HU$

11. The center detector is always located in the center of the IR at the central ray.

12. 200 mA

Chapter 7

Exercise I

1. A

2. D

3. A

4. C

5. C

6. D

7. B

8. C

9. A

10. B

11. D

12. B

13. C

14. A

15. D

16. C

17. C

Exercise 2

1. C

2. G

3. B

4. A

5. F

6. J

7. D

8. I

9. E

10. L

11. H

12. K

Exercise 3

1. Milliamperage (mA) and exposure time (seconds) are both directly proportional to the quantity of exposure.

2. Milliampere-seconds (mAs) are directly proportional to the total quantity of exposure and are used to indicate it.

3. 300 mA × 0.3 sec = 90 mAs

4. The mAs should be reduced to make the image lighter. This could be accomplished by reducing either the mA or the time. Time is usually the factor that is altered.

5. A short scale of contrast (obtained with lower kVp) provides greater differences between tissue densities that are similar; that is, greater contrast. A short scale of contrast is more desirable.

6. The standard mA and exposure time must be changed. An increase in mA followed with a corresponding decrease in exposure time to maintain mAs and density, will significantly reduce motion.

7. The scale of contrast is too long (the kVp is too high).
   Fog is causing decreased contrast. This could be due to fog from any source.

8. Increased SID or decreased focal spot size, or both, would improve the image.

9. Image blur affects the radiographic image sharpness or recorded detail. A shorter exposure time might solve the problem.

10. Maintain a stable position.
    Use positioning aids for comfort, such as radiolucent sponges.
    Use positioning aids for stability, such as sandbags or a table restraint.
    Provide clear instruction with ample time to comply.
    Use a shorter exposure time.

11. Film type
    Processing chemicals
    Tissue density
    kVp

12. OID
    SID
    Alignment of the part, central ray, or IR
    Central ray angulation, direction and degree of angulation

13. Geometric factors (increase in SID, decrease in OID)
    Reduction of motion
    Reduction of quantum mottle
    Use of the small focal spot
    Ensuring that intensifying screen contact is maintained

Chapter 8

Exercise I

1. A

2. A

3. B

4. A

5. A

6. B

7. C

8. D

9. C

10. B

11. D

12. D

13. B

14. C

15. A

16. D

Exercise 2

1. T

2. F

3. F

4. T

5. T

6. T

7. T

8. T

9. F

10. F

11. F

12. T

Exercise 3

1. The lead foil layer absorbs backscatter, preventing it from fogging the film. It is located between the back of the cassette and the back intensifying screen.

2. Damage to the frame may change its shape, preventing the screens from lying flat. This causes poor film/screen contact.
   Damage to the foam padding layer may prevent the screens from pressing tightly against the film, causing poor film/screen contact.

Damage to latches or hinges may prevent the cassette from closing tightly, causing exposure from light leaks.

3. Fast screens have larger phosphor crystals and thicker crystal layers, and may have a reflective layer. They require less exposure but do not provide the greatest image sharpness. Detail screens have small phosphor crystals and thinner crystal layers. They provide greater image sharpness than fast screens but require more exposure.

4. Blue (or blue-violet) and green (or yellow-green)

5. Determine, if possible, which cassette was used to expose the film and take it to the darkroom. If you cannot determine which cassette was used, take all cassettes of that size. Empty the cassette(s) and store the film in a light-tight box or in the film bin. Examine the cassette(s) for dirt, especially hair. Use a soft brush or compressed air from an aerosol can to remove the hair and any other dirt that may be present. Reload the cassette(s).

6. Aerosol can of compressed air
   Camel hair or sable hair brush
   Commercial screen cleaner recommended by manufacturer
   Soft, lint-free, disposable applicators such as nonwoven gauze squares

7. The weight of the boxes causes pressure. Film is sensitive to pressure and may become fogged.

8. Optimum temperature for film storage is 50° to 70° F (10° to 21° C).

9. Toe: base + fog level
   Straight line portion: film speed
   Straight line slope: contrast, latitude
   Shoulder: maximum density (D-max)

10. Film is made to be particularly sensitive to a specific portion of the electromagnetic spectrum. When screens are used with film that is not sensitive to the light given off by the screens, additional unnecessary exposure is required to produce an acceptable image. Incorrect matching of film and screens unnecessarily increases patient dose.

11. RS 50 to 100

12. *Latitude* is used to describe radiographic film along with contrast. *Latitude* is the term used when a wide range of densities can be recorded on the film. Latitude and contrast are inversely related. As the contrast of the film decreases, latitude increases.

A film with "wide latitude" will show many more densities than a film with high contrast. The term *low contrast* can be used instead of *wide latitude*.

Chapter 9

Exercise 1

1. E
2. B
3. G
4. A
5. F
6. D
7. C

Exercise 2

1. D
2. B
3. D
4. C
5. B
6. A
7. A
8. C

Exercise 3

1. Laser light
2. 10,000
3. Digital radiography (DR)
4. Ability to see images very fast

   A wide dynamic range is enabled

   Image density and contrast can easily be adjusted
5. Quantum mottle

6. Picture archiving and communications systems
7. Compensating filters
8. kVp
9. Covered with lead
10. Scatter radiation

Exercise 4

1. F
2. T
3. T
4. F
5. T

Chapter 10

Exercise 1

1. D
2. A
3. A
4. C
5. D
6. D
7. D
8. B
9. A
10. B
11. C
12. B
13. B
14. B
15. A

16. A

17. C

18. A

Exercise 2

1. Underreplenishment

2. Underreplenishment

3. Underreplenishment

4. Overreplenishment

5. Underreplenishment

6. Overreplenishment

Exercise 3

1. You might suspect an unsafe safelight if the base + fog level on a processor quality control film was higher than usual. You might also begin to suspect this if films showed a flat, gray appearance with exposures that usually produce good contrast. To determine the safety of the safelight, you would conduct a safelight test as instructed in this chapter using a presensitized film. If the test indicated that the safelight was not safe, you might move the light to a location more remote from the work area or replace the light bulb with one of lower wattage. You should also check the safelight filter to be sure that it is not damaged and that it is of the correct type for the film in use. Repeat the safelight test after corrective measures have been taken to be sure that these measures were adequate.

2. Information to be imprinted on the film should include at least the patient's name, an identifying number (file number, chart number, or birth date), the date of the examination, and the name and location of the x-ray facility.

3. The primary function of the developer is to change the exposed silver halide crystals into black metallic silver. The two functions of the fixer are to clear the film (remove any remaining silver halide crystals) and to tan (shrink and preserve) the emulsion.

4. The required fixing time is at least twice the clearing time. Note the time needed to clear the film and multiply this time by 2.

5. Water flow is less than adequate.
   Water tank is overcrowded.
   Film was in the fixer for an excessive period.

6. Developer replenisher must not only make up for lost solution volume, the replenisher must also compensate for lost strength in the solution that remains. Fixer replenisher needs to be much stronger than the original solution because solution is carried into the tank and out of it. Thus a small volume of replenisher must compensate for large changes in the strength of the solution.

7. The rate needs to be increased so that the processing of fewer films will bring sufficient replenishment to compensate for deterioration of the solutions during idle periods. The correct rates should be determined by calculating the approximate number of films processed per week and consulting the processor operation manual.

8. Increased fog and decreased contrast usually occur together. These results may be caused by outdated or improperly stored film, unsafe safelights, incorrect processor temperature, or failure to add starter when changing solutions. If the fog level is significantly high and the solutions have just been changed, lack of starter should be suspected. If that is not the case, check the expiration date on the film box and check the quality of the film by performing another sensitometric test in total darkness. If the film does not appear to be fogged when processed in darkness, perform a safelight safety test.

9. To clean up a chemical spill, first restrict access to the area and consult the material safety data sheet on file for the chemical. For cleaning up a fixer spill, you will need cleaning supplies (bucket, sponge, and mop), a protective apron, splash-proof goggles, and nitrile gloves. If you get some in your eye, you should proceed to an eyewash station and rinse the eye thoroughly. If no eyewash station is available, place the eye under gently running water for several minutes. If pain persists, see a physician.

Chapter 11

Exercise 1

1. C

2. D

3. B

4. D

5. A

6. A

7. B

8. A

9. A

10. C

11. D

12. B

13. A

14. C

15. D

16. A

Exercise 2

1. T

2. T

3. F

4. F

5. F

6. F

7. T

8. T

9. T

10. T

11. F

12. T

13. T

14. F

Exercise 3

1. Photoelectric interactions produce characteristic scatter radiation.

2. Part thickness
   Field size

3. The quantity of fog is increased because the scatter produced with higher kVp has greater energy.

4. The patient is the principal source of scattered radiation fog in radiography.

5. Typically a table Bucky for general use has a ratio of 12:1.

6. The usual minimum frequency for stationary grids is 103 lines/inch in permanent installations with ratios of 10:1 or 12:1.

7. A 35 × 43 cm IR will show normal radiographic density in the center and decreased density with lengthwise streaks and apparent grid lines on both sides.

8. The lateral projection of the cervical spine

9. A "spot film" shows increased image quality because of the reduction of scattered radiation fog. Recorded detail will also be improved because of the decrease in distortion that results when the area of clinical interest is centered to the central ray.

10. Usually this is determined by referring to the technique chart, because this chart will indicate grid use when the average adult part size is sufficient to require a grid. When in doubt, measure the part and use a grid if the part measures 10 to 12 cm or greater.

Chapter 12

Exercise 1

1. D

2. C

3. C

4. B

5. A

6. B

7. D

8. A

9. A

10. D

11. C

12. C

13. B

14. D

15. D

16. True

17. False

18. True

Exercise 2

1. 100 mAs

2. 7.5 mAs

3. 400 mAs

4. 100 mAs

5. 25 mAs

Exercise 3

1. ↑

2. ↑

3. ↓

4. ↓

5. ↑

6. ↓

7. ↑

8. ↓

9. ↓

10. ↓

11. ↑

12. ↓

13. ↑

14. ↓

Exercise 4

1. From Appendix B: 300 mA, 0.035 sec, 120 kVp, 72 inches SID, and 10:1 grid, using RS 300 screens and XYZ film

2. An x-ray caliper is used to measure body part thickness in units of centimeters (cm).

3. Change processing solutions.
   Check processor performance for several days to be certain that performance is stable.
   Check local radiation control regulations to determine what information must be included on the chart.
   Obtain the necessary tools. Depending on the method you plan to use, you may need an internally consistent chart from another facility, a Supertech calculator, a radiographic phantom, or an appointment with your film company's technical representative.

4. AP cervical spine: 70 to 80 kVp
   AP thoracic spine: 80 to 90 kVp
   AP lumbar spine: 74 to 88 kVp

5. Elbow: 50 or 100 mA to use the small focal spot
   Lumbar spine: 200 mA for relatively fast exposure without taxing the tube
   Chest: 300 mA for shortest possible exposure time to prevent image blur from involuntary motion of the heart

6. 10 mAs ÷ 100 mA = ¹⁄₁₀ (or 0.1) sec

7. Conditions requiring an increase:
   Chest conditions: atelectasis, bronchiectasis, carcinoma (advanced), edema (pulmonary), empyema, hydropneumothorax, pleural effusion, pneumoconiosis diseases, pneumonia, thoracoplasty, tuberculosis (calcific and military)
   Conditions of bone: acromegaly, arthritis (rheumatoid), Charcot joint, osteochondroma, osteomyelitis (healed), osteopetrosis, Paget disease
   Abdominal conditions: ascites, cirrhosis of liver
   Soft tissue conditions: edema
   Generalized conditions: heavy musculature, large bones
   Casts and splints: wet plaster cast, dry plaster cast, aluminum splint
   Conditions requiring a decrease:
   Chest conditions: chronic obstructive pulmonary disease (COPD, emphysema), pneumothorax, tuberculosis (active)
   Conditions of bone: arthritis (degenerative), gout, hyperparathyroidism, metastasis (lytic), multiple myeloma, necrosis osteomyelitis (active), osteoporosis, sarcoma, syphilis (advanced)

Abdominal conditions: bowel obstruction, pneumoperitoneum
Generalized conditions: advanced age, atrophy, emaciation

8. Increased latitude and decreased dose are obtained by increasing kVp. To change kVp without altering radiographic density, the 15% rule is used (increase kVp by 15% and divide mAs by 2). The new exposure is 200 mA, 0.15 sec, and 81 kVp.

9. The formula needed here is $mAs_1/mAs_2 = SID_1^2/SID_2^2$. The result is 6.17 mAs.

10. This could be accomplished by reducing either the kVp or the mAs. To compensate with kVp, subtract 14 kVp: 76 kVp - 14 kVp = 62 kVp. To compensate with mAs, divide original mAs by 2.5: 10 mAs ÷ 2.5 = 4 mAs.

Chapter 13

Exercise 1

1. B
2. A
3. C
4. C
5. D
6. D
7. A
8. A
9. B
10. C
11. D
12. B
13. C
14. A
15. C
16. B
17. C

18. B
19. D
20. C
21. False
22. True
23. True
24. False

Exercise 2

1. B
2. F
3. E
4. H
5. G
6. J
7. I
8. C
9. D
10. A
11. K

Exercise 3

1. R = Coulombs per kilogram (C/kg)
   rad = Gray
   rem = Sievert

2.

1 rad x-ray	1 rad × 1 (W_R)	=	1 rem
1 rad thermal neutrons	1 rad × 5 (W_R)	=	5 rem
<u>1 rad fast neutrons</u>	1 rad × 20 (W_R)	=	<u>20 rem</u>
3 rad total dose	total dose	=	26 rem

3. From the graph, an exposure at 80 kVp and 60 inches SSD results in an exposure rate of 3 mR/mAs; 3 mR/mAs × 20 mAs = 60 mR entrance skin exposure.

4. Long-term (latent) effects usually occur 5 to 30 years after exposure. They are stochastic (random and unpredictable) and the severity is not related

to dose. They include malignant diseases, such as cancer and leukemia. Short-term effects result from higher doses and are nonstochastic. They include loss of function of organs and tissue, especially blood cells; and syndromes, such as radiation sickness and central nervous system effects, which involves seizures, coma, and death. The severity of short-term effects is directly related to dose.

5. Although all radiation exposure involves some degree of risk, the technology we use today permits us to do examinations like this with very small amounts of radiation and extremely low risk. The possibility of any bad effect from this examination is less than 1 in a million. You took a much greater risk today when you drove from your home to the clinic. It is also important to consider the benefit of the examination and the possible risks involved in failing to get the information this examination will provide.

6. At a dose of 25 rem, you would see blood changes. Death would occur at an acute dose of 600 rem.

7. Gonad shielding should be used on all patients under age 55 when the reproductive organs are in or near the primary x-ray beam and when the shield will not interfere with the purpose of the examination. The shield must be equal to 0.5 mm lead equivalent. The purpose of gonad shielding is to decrease the risk of genetic mutations that could have negative effects on future generations.

8. Double-check the requisition and the patient identification.
Explain the procedure and obtain the patient's cooperation.
Use established procedures for film placement, tube placement, and patient positioning to prevent overlooking details.
Collimate to include only the anatomic area of clinical interest.
Shield gonads and any sensitive organs near the radiation field.
Measure the patient correctly and check the technique chart precisely.
Consider whether any variations in the usual technique are needed for this particular patient.
Be certain that the processor is operating correctly and use standard procedures for processing.
Maintain equipment, processor, and accessories in good condition.
Use low-dose techniques.

9. Low-dose techniques involve using optimum kVp (the highest kVp consistent with acceptable contrast), the fastest screens and film that are consistent with

acceptable definition, a minimum SID of 40 inches, and nongrid techniques when appropriate.

10. Be sure that a policy exists for this purpose and that you are familiar with it. Possible considerations include posting warning signs and discussing the possibility of pregnancy with female patients of childbearing age. Neither the 10-day rule nor an early pregnancy test can guarantee that the patient is not pregnant, but these can greatly decrease the likelihood of pregnancy.

11. The shielding provided by the control booth.

12. The effective dose (EfD) limit for nonpregnant workers over the age of 18 is 5 rem per year. The DE limit for pregnant workers is 10% of the annual limit (0.5 rem) over the 9-month course of the pregnancy. The ALARA principle is used in conjunction with both limits. Even when exposures are well below DE limits, they should be reduced further if it is reasonably achievable.

13. As Low As Reasonably Achievable

14. Ionizing radiation is radiation that, when passing through the body, produces positively and negatively charged particles.

15. Radiation protection is the measures taken to safeguard patients, personnel, and the public from unnecessary exposure to ionizing radiation.

16. Radiation badges should be worn in the region of the collar and on the anterior surface of the body. They should be on the outside of the lead apron when an apron is worn when holding patients or during fluoroscopy.

Chapter 14

Exercise 1

1. C

2. D

3. C

4. D

5. C

6. A

7. B

8. A

9. D

10. C

Exercise 2

1. C

2. K

3. E

4. I

5. G

6. A

7. D

8. B

9. H

10. F

11. J

Exercise 3

Top row, left to right:

1. Greenstick

2. Spiral

3. Overriding

4. Comminuted

Bottom row, left to right:

5. Transverse

6. Compression

7. Depressed

8. Avulsion

Exercise 4

1. Plasma membrane
   Cytoplasm
   Nucleus

2. Bone
   Cartilage
   Fat

3. Groups of similar cells that work together to perform a common function are called *tissues*, whereas an *organ* is a group of tissues that act together to perform a special function.

4. Respiratory: nose, mouth, pharynx, larynx, trachea, bronchi, bronchioles, and lungs
   Digestive: mouth, teeth, tongue, salivary glands, pharynx, esophagus, stomach, small intestine, large intestine, appendix, rectum and anal canal, liver, gallbladder, and pancreas
   Urinary: kidneys, ureters, bladder, and urethra

5. The skeletal system provides a ridged framework for the body.

6. The outer portion is the cortex. The inner portion is spongy bone, which may also be called *cancellous bone*.

7. Synarthrosis: joints of the skull
   Amphiarthrosis: intervertebral joints, sacroiliac joints, pubic symphysis
   Diarthrosis: all freely moveable joints—hip, knee, shoulder, elbow, wrist, etc.

8. Abduct: move away from center of body
   Adduct: move toward center of body
   Extend: straighten a hinge joint, straighten the spine (bend backward)
   Flex: bend a hinge joint, bend the spine forward
   Pronate: rotate the forearm so the palm of the hand faces down
   Supinate: rotate the forearm so the palm of the hand faces up

9. Elbow

10. Left lateral position

11. Anteroposterior (AP)

12. Left lateral projection

13. Chest respiration: inspiration
    Abdominal respiration: expiration

14. Crosswise

15. Endogenous: stroke, heart attack, scurvy, rickets, pellagra, goiter, rheumatoid arthritis, lupus erythematosus, and ankylosing spondylitis

Exogenous: fracture, dislocation, soft tissue injury, infection

16. Swelling
Reddening
Heat at the site
Pain

17. Acute conditions are characterized by sudden onset, whereas chronic conditions are of long duration. Benign conditions are lesions that are limited in growth and remain at one site, whereas malignant conditions are cancers that grow more rapidly, invade surrounding structures, and can spread (metastasize) to distant sites

18. *-itis:* inflammatory conditions
-oma: neoplasms or tumors; can be benign or malignant

Chapter 15

Exercise 1

1. C

2. B

3. C

4. D

5. C

6. A

7. C

8. D

9. D

10. D

11. C

12. A

13. B

14. C

15. B

16. C

Exercise 2

Fig. 15-1
1. Distal phalanx
2. Middle phalanx
3. Proximal phalanx
4. Distal phalanx
5. Proximal phalanx
6. Capitate
7. Trapezium
8. Trapezoid
9. Scaphoid
10. Lunate
11. Triquetrum
12. Pisiform
13. Hamate
14. Metacarpals
15. Phalanges

Fig. 15-2
1. Head
2. Neck
3. Tuberosity
4. Styloid
5. Styloid
6. Head
7. Shaft
8. Coronoid (process)
9. Semilunar notch
10. Olecranon (process)
11. Shaft
12. Styloid
13. Head
14. Neck
15. Head
16. Coronoid (process)
17. Semilunar notch

Fig. 15-3
1. Greater tubercle
2. Lesser tubercle
3. Shaft
4. Lateral epicondyle
5. Capitulum
6. Coronoid fossa
7. Trochlea
8. Medial epicondyle
9. Head
10. Head
11. Shaft
12. Capitulum
13. Trochlea
14. Medial epicondyle

Fig. 15-4

1. Scapular notch
2. Medial angle
3. Inferior angle
4. Glenoid process
5. Glenoid fossa
6. Acromion
7. Coracoid process
8. Acromion
9. Glenoid fossa
10. Glenoid process
11. Inferior angle
12. Supraspinatus fossa
13. Medial angle
14. Scapular notch
15. Medial angle
16. Coracoid process
17. Glenoid fossa
18. Anterior surface
19. Inferior angle
20. Posterior surface
21. Axillary border
22. Acromion

Fig. 15-5

1. Acromial extremity
2. Sternal extremity
3. Shaft

Fig. 15-6

1. Medial end of clavicle
2. Coracoid process
3. Inferior angle of scapula
4. Medial epicondyle
5. Ulnar styloid process
6. Olecranon process of ulna
7. Radial styloid process
8. Lateral epicondyle
9. Greater tubercle
10. Acromion process

Exercise 3

1. The middle bone of the third digit is the middle phalanx of the third digit. The carpal bone that articulates with the first metacarpal is the trapezium.

2. The ulna is medial to the radius.

3. Radial head
   Trochlear notch (ulna)
   Capitulum (lateral humerus)
   Trochlea (medial humerus)

4. Acromion process
   Coracoid process

Spine of the scapula
Inferior angle

5. For the thumb, the AP projection is preferred to the PA projection.
   The thumb is oblique when the hand is pronated, but the fingers are in the PA position.
   Examination of the thumb must include the entire first metacarpal, but examinations of the fingers need only include a portion of their respective metacarpals.

6. The fingers are extended for a PA projection of the hand, but they are flexed into a loose fist for a PA projection of the wrist. The hand projection is centered at the third MP joint, whereas the wrist is centered midway between the styloid processes.

7. Ulnar deviation
   Stecher method

8. A routine shoulder examination consists of two AP projections, one with the humerus in internal rotation and one with external rotation. Examination for acute injury includes an AP projection with no rotation of the humerus and a transthoracic lateral projection. The trauma views are designed to show the humerus in two projections at right angles to each other without rotating the injured arm, which could cause both extreme pain and further injury.

9. A routine clavicle study consists of PA and axial projections to place the clavicle as close to the film as possible. If the patient is recumbent, a supine position may be more comfortable and AP and AP axial projections would be performed.

10. Positioning the arm behind the back gives a superior view of the acromion and coracoid processes but sometimes results in superimposition of the humerus over the body of the scapula. Positioning the arm overhead provides an unobstructed view of the body, but the humeral head superimposes the superior structures of the scapula. Positioning the arm across the chest also compromises visualization of the superior structures but is often the only position attainable by the patient with a scapular injury.

11. Mentioned in the text were boxer's fracture (fifth metacarpal), occult fracture of the scaphoid, Colles fracture (distal radius), Monteggia fracture (ulnar fracture with radial head displacement), radial head fracture, and clavicle fracture.

12. Bursitis
    Tendonitis
    Osteoarthritis

Osteomyelitis
Bone cyst
Bone infarct
Neoplastic and metastatic disease (both osteolytic and osteoblastic)

Exercise 4

Fig. 15-7
1. Phalanges
2. Carpals
3. Radius
4. Ulna
5. Metacarpals

Fig. 15-8
1. Phalanges
2. Metacarpals
3. Carpal bones
4. Radius
5. Ulna

Fig. 15-9
1. Trapezoid
2. Scaphoid
3. Radial styloid
4. Radius
5. Ulna
6. Ulnar styloid
7. Lunate
8. Triquetrum
9. Capitate

Fig. 15-10
1. First metacarpal
2. Trapezium
3. Scaphoid
4. Radius
5. Ulna

Fig. 15-11
1. Fifth metacarpal
2. Hamate
3. Pisiform
4. Scaphoid
5. Lunate
6. Distal radius
7. Distal ulna
8. Distal radius

Fig. 15-12
1. Hamulus of hamate
2. Pisiform
3. Trapezium
4. Capitate

Fig. 15-13
1. Ulna
2. Radius

Fig. 15-14
1. Ulna
2. Radius

Fig. 15-15
1. Medial epicondyle
2. Olecranon process
3. Radial head
4. Capitulum
5. Lateral epicondyle
6. Olecranon fossa

Fig. 15-16
1. Radial head
2. Olecranon process
3. Distal humerus
4. Coronoid process

Fig. 15-17
1. Capitulum
2. Radial head

Fig. 15-18
1. Humeral head
2. Shaft of humerus
3. Lateral epicondyle
4. Medial epicondyle
5. Body of scapula
6. Humeral head
7. Shaft of humerus
8. Olecranon process
9. Body of scapula

Fig. 15-19
1. Coracoid process
2. Glenoid process
3. Shaft of humerus
4. Humeral head
5. Greater tubercle
6. Acromion
7. Distal clavicle

Fig. 15-20
1. Proximal end of clavicle
2. Coracoid process
3. Humeral head
4. Acromion
5. Acromioclavicular joint
6. Distal end of clavicle

Fig. 15-21
1. Scapular spine
2. Medial (vertebral) border
3. Coracoid process
4. Body
5. Inferior angle
6. Lateral border
7. Glenoid fossa
8. Acromion

Chapter 16

Exercise 1

1. B

2. D

3. C

4. A

5. A

6. D

7. C

8. A

9. B

10. D

11. B

12. C

13. B

14. D

15. B

16. A

Exercise 2

1. Great toe: two phalanges
   Second toe: three phalanges

2. The fibula is lateral to the tibia.

3. The knee joint is formed by the articulation between the femur and the tibia.

4. Iliac crest
   Anterior superior iliac spine (ASIS)
   Symphysis pubis
   Ischial tuberosity

5. The knee is flexed for the AP foot projection; it is extended for the AP ankle projection.
   The plantar surface of the foot is in contact with the IR for an AP foot projection; the posterior surface of the heel is in contact with the IR for an AP ankle projection.
   The central ray is angled toward the heel for the AP foot projection; the central ray is perpendicular to the IR for the AP ankle projection.
   The foot is everted for the oblique foot projection; the entire leg is rotated medially for the oblique ankle projection.

6. The entire leg is medially rotated so that the sagittal plane of the foot and leg forms an angle of 15 to 25 degrees with the vertical plane. A line between the malleoli is parallel to the film. The ankle is dorsiflexed so that long axis of the foot forms 90 degrees with the long axis of the lower leg.

7. The intercondylar fossa or "tunnel" projections: Holmblad and Camp-Coventry methods
   Tangential projection of the patella or "sunrise" view: Settegast method

8. PA and lateral projections should be taken. Take care not to flex the knee more than 10 degrees.

9. A routine hip study includes AP (with medial rotation) and frog-leg lateral projections of the hip region. Examination for possible hip fracture begins with an AP projection of the entire pelvis and both hips. The hips are not rotated from their presenting position. The initial examination is taken without rotating the hips because rotation could cause displacement or further injury if there is a hip fracture. The entire pelvis is taken because the injury could be to the pelvis itself. If this is the case, the entire pelvis must be evaluated because it is common for pelvis fractures to occur in pairs. The axiolateral projection is performed instead of the frog-leg lateral. This projection is taken without moving or rotating the affected leg.

10. Stress fracture is a simple, nondisplaced fracture that occurs from repeated traumatic injury. Stress fractures are common in the metatarsals and in the calcaneus as a result of running, jogging, or marching. They also occur in the tibia, fibula, femoral shaft, femoral neck, ischium, and pubis.

Bimalleolar fracture involves the malleoli of the distal fibula and the distal medial tibia.
Spiral fracture of the tibia encircles the bone in a spiral pattern and is usually caused by a twisting injury.
Hip fracture may occur to the head of the femur, the femoral neck, or the intertrochanteric region.

11. Arthritic conditions: rheumatoid arthritis, osteo-arthritis, gout (especially common in the great toe)
Osteomyelitis
Neoplastic and metastatic bone disease

Exercise 3

Fig. 16-1
1. Distal phalanx
2. Middle phalanx
3. Proximal phalanx
4. Lateral cuneiform
5. Cuboid
6. Calcaneus
7. Talus
8. Navicular
9. Intermediate cuneiform
10. Medial cuneiform
11. Metatarsals
12. Phalanges
13. Talus
14. Calcaneus
15. Medial cuneiform
16. First metatarsal
17. Phalanges
18. Navicular

Fig. 16-2
1. Intercondylar eminences
2. Medial condyle
3. Tibial tuberosity
4. Tibia
5. Shafts
6. Medial malleolus
7. Lateral malleolus
8. Fibula
9. Head
10. Styloid
11. Lateral condyle

Fig. 16-3
1. Tibia
2. Medial malleolus
3. Talus
4. Lateral malleolus
5. Fibula

Fig. 16-4
1. Head
2. Greater trochanter
3. Shaft
4. Lateral condyle
5. Medial condyle
6. Medial epicondyle
7. Lesser trochanter
8. Neck
9. Head
10. Neck
11. Lesser trochanter
12. Shaft
13. Medial epicondyle
14. Medial condyle
15. Intercondylar fossa
16. Lateral condyle
17. Lateral epicondyle
18. Intertrochanteric crest
19. Greater trochanter
20. Lateral condyle
21. Intercondylar fossa
22. Medial condyle
23. Base
24. Apex

Fig. 16-5
1. Ilium
2. Pubis
3. Ischium
4. Pubic arch
5. Brim of the lesser pelvis
6. Sacroiliac joints
7. Ilium
8. Arcuate line
9. Acetabulum
10. Pubic symphysis
11. Coccyx
12. Sacrum

Fig. 16-6
1. Phalanges
2. Metatarsals
3. Medial cuneiform
4. Intermediate cuneiform
5. Lateral cuneiform
6. Navicular
7. Talus
8. Cuboid

Fig. 16-7
1. Cuboid
2. Calcaneus
3. Talus
4. Navicular
5. Cuneiforms

Fig. 16-8
1. First metatarsal
2. Proximal phalanx
3. Distal phalanx

Fig. 16-9
1. Calcaneocuboid articulation
2. Calcaneus
3. Talus
4. Calcaneus

Fig. 16-10
1. Distal tibia
2. Medial malleolus
3. Talus
4. Lateral malleolus
5. Distal fibula

Fig. 16-11
1. Distal fibula
2. Distal tibia
3. Calcaneus
4. Navicular
5. Talus

Fig. 16-12
1. Tibia
2. Fibula
3. Fibula
4. Tibia

Fig. 16-13
1. Distal femur
2. Medial epicondyle
3. Tibial plateau
4. Proximal tibia
5. Head of fibula
6. Intercondylar eminences
7. Lateral epicondyle
8. Patella

Fig. 16-14
1. Distal femur
2. Patella
3. Lateral condyle
4. Medial condyle
5. Fibula
6. Tibia

Fig 16-15
1. Greater trochanter
2. Lesser trochanter
3. Shaft of femur
4. Femoral neck
5. Femoral head

6. Acetabulum
7. Femoral head
8. Lesser trochanter
9. Shaft of femur

Fig. 16-16
1. L5
2. Sacroiliac joint
3. Sacrum
4. Femoral head
5. Pubis
6. Pubic symphysis
7. Ischium
8. Lesser trochanter
9. Greater trochanter
10. Femoral neck
11. Acetabulum
12. Anterior superior iliac spine
13. Ilium
14. Iliac crest

Fig. 16-17
1. Ilium
2. Acetabulum
3. Femoral head
4. Greater trochanter
5. Femoral neck
6. Ischium
7. Pubis

Chapter 17

Exercise 1

1. C

2. D

3. A

4. C

5. B

6. D

7. C

8. B

9. B

10. B

11. C

12. D

13. B

14. D

15. B

16. D

17. A

18. A

19. B

20. D

Exercise 2

1. Cervical spine: 7 vertebrae
   Thoracic spine: 12 vertebrae
   Lumbar spine: 5 vertebrae
   Sacrum: 5 segments
   Coccyx: 4 segments

2. The cervical and lumbar spines have a lordotic curve
   The thoracic spine has a kyphotic curve.
   The sacrum and coccyx together form a kyphotic curve.

3. The atlas has no body and its superior articular processes are set at a different angle than the superior articular processes of the other cervical vertebrae. The axis has a superior projection from the body, called the *dens*, that passes through the ring of the atlas. The atlas is capable of rotation on the axis. This is a far greater degree of rotation than is possible between any of the other vertebral bodies.

4. Mental point: inferior midportion of the lower jaw
   Mastoid process: bony projection behind the earlobe
   Angle of mandible: "corner" of the lower jaw beneath the ear lobe
   Laryngeal prominence: "Adam's apple" in the center of the anterior neck
   Jugular (sternal) notch: U-shaped bony structure at the base of the throat

5. Extend the neck so that the line between the occlusal surface of the upper teeth and the base of the occipital bone is parallel to the floor.

6. Left cervical intervertebral foramina: left anterior oblique or right posterior oblique
   Cervical zygapophyseal joints: lateral projection

Lumbar intervertebral foramina: lateral projection
Left lumbar zygapophyseal joints: left posterior oblique or right anterior oblique
Sacroiliac (SI) joints: AP axial projection of the lumbosacral joint and/or posterior oblique position—left posterior oblique for right SI joint and right posterior oblique for left SI joint

7. The lateral projection in the neutral position should be processed and shown to the physician before proceeding with the flexion and extension positions. If there is an unstable cervical spine fracture, these positions could cause subluxation of the spinal vertebra, placing pressure on the spinal cord and risking paralysis or death.

8. This is often caused by failure to take the anode heel effect into account and placing the patient's head toward the anode end of the x-ray tube. If the position were correct for use of the anode heel effect, a wedge filter could be used to reduce the exposure to the upper thoracic area. Increasing kVp, according to the 15% rule, would also result in a more uniform density by reducing contrast and increasing penetration of the lower thoracic area.

9. The patient should be instructed to disrobe except for underpants and put on a gown. Specifically, her bra must be removed. Shoes should be removed for upright examinations.

10. Cervical ribs: riblike structures attached to C7
    Lumbar ribs: riblike structures attached to L1
    Sacralization of L5: fusion between one or both transverse processes of L5 and the sacrum
    Lumbarization of S1: failure of the first sacral segment to fuse with the body of the sacrum
    Six lumbar vertebrae: an extra lumbar vertebra occurring in the presence of the proper number of segments in the other sections of the spine
    Spina bifida occulta: failure of the posterior elements of a vertebra to fuse and form a solid vertebral arch

11. Compression fractures with wedging of midthoracic vertebral bodies are common among older women with osteoporosis.

12. Hypertrophic arthritic changes, such as bony spurs on the vertebrae, may cause stenosis (narrowing) of the intervertebral foramina.
    Misalignment of vertebrae, subluxation, or spondylolisthesis may cause crowding of the nerve pathways.
    Disk herniation is also a common cause of nerve root compression.

Exercise 3

Fig. 17-1
1. Lordotic curve
2. Kyphotic curve
3. Lordotic curve
4. Kyphotic curve

Fig. 17-2
1. Posterior arch
2. Transverse process
3. Superior articular process
4. Transverse atlantal ligament
5. Anterior arch
6. Lateral mass
7. Transverse foramen

Fig. 17-3
1. Dens (odontoid process)
2. Transverse process
3. Inferior articular process
4. Facet
5. Superior articular process
6. Facet
7. Dens (odontoid process)
8. Body
9. Transverse foramen
10. Transverse process
11. Vertebral notch
12. Facet
13. Inferior articular process
14. Spinous process
15. Lamina
16. Superior articular process

Fig. 17-4
1. Spinous process (bifid)
2. Vertebral foramen
3. Transverse foramen
4. Body
5. Pedicle
6. Transverse process
7. Superior articular process
8. Lamina
9. Articular pillar
10. Body
11. Transverse process
12. Vertebral notch
13. Inferior articular process
14. Spinous process
15. Lamina
16. Superior articular process

Fig. 17-5
1. Spinous process
2. Lamina

3. Transverse process
4. Vertebral foramen
5. Superior costal facet
6. Body
7. Pedicle
8. Costal facet (for tubercle of rib)
9. Superior articular process and facet
10. Pedicle
11. Superior costal facet (demifacet)
12. Inferior costal facet (demifacet)
13. Inferior vertebral notch
14. Inferior articular process
15. Spinous process
16. Lamina
17. Transverse process
18. Facet for costal tubercle
19. Superior articular process

Fig. 17-6
1. Spinous process
2. Lamina
3. Mammillary process
4. Transverse process
5. Vertebral foramen
6. Body
7. Pedicle
8. Superior articular process
9. Accessory process
10. Pars interarticularis
11. Superior vertebral notch
12. Pedicle
13. Inferior vertebral notch
14. Inferior articular process
15. Facet
16. Lamina
17. Spinous process
18. Transverse process
19. Superior articular process

Fig. 17-7
1. Sacral promontory
2. Base
3. Body of sacral segment
4. Pelvic sacral foramina
5. Apex
6. Base
7. Apex
8. Coccyx
9. Sacrum
10. Superior articular process
11. Base
12. Promontory
13. Articular surface (sacroiliac joint)
14. Sacrum
15. Coccyx
16. Coccygeal cornu
17. Sacral cornu

Fig. 17-8
1. Mandible
2. Axis (C2)
3. C7
4. Occipital base

Fig. 17-9
1. C4-C5 zygapophyseal joint
2. Spinous process of C7
3. Trachea
4. Body of C3
5. Anterior arch of atlas (C1)

Fig. 17-10
1. L1
2. Iliac crest
3. Sacrum

Fig. 17-11
1. Sacrum
2. Lumbosacral joint
3. Body of L3

Fig. 17-12
1. Lumbosacral joint
2. Sacroiliac joint

Chapter 18

Exercise 1

1. C
2. B
3. B
4. D
5. C
6. A
7. D
8. C
9. B
10. C
11. D
12. A
13. D

14. A
15. A
16. C
17. D
18. B
19. B
20. D

Exercise 2

1. Manubrium: upper portion, just below the jugular (sternal) notch
   Body (gladiolus): the long central portion between the breasts
   Xiphoid process: the lower tip of the sternum just above the solar plexus

2. Drawing of a lung:

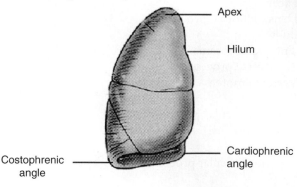

Apex
Hilum
Cardiophrenic angle
Costophrenic angle

3. Esophagus: digestive system
   Trachea: respiratory system
   Heart: circulatory system
   Thymus gland: lymphatic system

4. Right upper quadrant: liver, gallbladder, colon (hepatic flexure)
   Left upper quadrant: stomach, spleen, colon (splenic flexure)
   Right lower quadrant: cecum, appendix, small intestine
   Left lower quadrant: sigmoid colon, small intestine

5. Left upper anterior ribs: PA, RAO
   Right lower posterior ribs: AP, RPO

6. Ribs below the diaphragm should be exposed on expiration to raise the diaphragm and see as many ribs as possible below the diaphragm.

7. Rib radiography usually involves only one side of the chest; chest radiography includes both sides.
Rib radiography may be done recumbent or upright; chest radiography should always be done upright, if possible.
Rib radiography is done at 40 inches SID; chest radiography is done at 72 inches SID.
Rib radiography is done in the 70- to 80-kVp range to prevent overpenetrating the ribs; chest radiography is done with high kVp (100 to 130) to provide latitude and to penetrate the ribs and the mediastinum.
Rib studies include frontal and oblique views. The exact projections are selected to best visualize the area of injury. Chest radiography includes PA and left lateral projections to demonstrate the lungs and to minimize magnification of the cardiac shadow.

8. If a patient with acute abdominal pain cannot stand for an upright AP abdomen, a left lateral decubitus projection should be taken. This is important to demonstrate possible fluid levels and intraperitoneal air that cannot be seen except with a horizontal x-ray beam.

9. Bacterial pneumonia
Viral pneumonia
Aspiration pneumonia

10. Cardiac enlargement
Pleural edema
Pleural effusion

11. Distention of the small bowel with excessive gas is typically seen in cases of bowel obstruction. Air-fluid levels are seen on projections taken with a horizontal x-ray beam.

12. Abdominal pain may be caused by a pathologic condition of the lower lungs or the diaphragm that can only be seen on chest radiographs. If there is free intraperitoneal air because of the rupture of a hollow viscus, it is often better seen on chest radiographs than on abdominal films.

Exercise 3

Fig. 18-1
1. Jugular notch
2. Clavicular notch
3. Manubrium
4. Sternal angle
5. Body
6. Xiphoid process
7. Costal cartilage
8. Ribs

Fig. 18-2
1. Jugular notch
2. Clavicle
3. Manubrium
4. Sternal angle
5. Body
6. Xiphoid process

Fig. 18-3
1. Trachea
2. Arch of aorta
3. Lung
4. Diaphragm

Fig. 18-4
1. Cardiac notch
2. Apex
3. Superior lobe
4. Oblique fissure
5. Inferior lobe
6. Costophrenic angle
7. Cardiophrenic angles
8. Costophrenic angles
9. Oblique fissure
10. Inferior lobe
11. Middle lobe
12. Horizontal fissure
13. Superior lobe
14. Apex

Fig. 18-5
1. Left primary bronchus
2. Terminal bronchiole
3. Alveolar duct
4. Alveolus
5. Alveolar sac
6. Carina
7. Pleural space
8. Pleura
9. Right primary bronchus
10. Bronchiole
11. Trachea
12. Larynx

Fig. 18-6
1. Left upper
2. Left lower
3. Right lower
4. Right upper

Fig. 18-7
1. Right hypochondriac region
2. Epigastric region
3. Left hypochondriac region
4. Right lumbar region
5. Umbilical region

6. Left lumbar region
7. Right iliac (inguinal) region
8. Hypogastric region
9. Left iliac (inguinal) region

Fig. 18-8
1. Esophagus
2. Liver, left lobe
3. Stomach
4. Spleen
5. Pancreas
6. Splenic flexure
7. Transverse colon
8. Small intestine
9. Descending colon
10. Sigmoid colon
11. Urinary bladder
12. Appendix
13. Ileum
14. Ascending colon
15. Gallbladder
16. Liver, right lobe
17. Diaphragm
18. Falciform ligament

Exercise 4

Fig. 18-9
1. First rib
2. Anterior second rib
3. Posterior tenth rib

Fig. 18-10
1. Diaphragm
2. Eleventh rib
3. Eighth rib

Fig. 18-11
1. Xiphoid process
2. Body of sternum
3. Sternal angle
4. Manubrium

Fig. 18-12
1. Manubrium
2. Body of sternum
3. Xiphoid tip

Fig. 18-13
1. Clavicle
2. Aortic knob
3. Left hilum
4. Heart
5. Costophrenic angle
6. Right hilum

7. Apex
8. Trachea

Fig. 18-14
1. Lung apices
2. Aortic arch
3. Heart
4. Dome of diaphragm
5. Costophrenic angles

Fig. 18-15
1. Intestinal gas shadows
2. Left kidney
3. Psoas muscle margin
4. Intestinal gas shadows
5. Liver

Fig. 18-16
1. Kidneys
2. Psoas muscle margin
3. Gas in colon
4. Liver margin

Chapter 19

Exercise 1

1. C

2. B

3. C

4. A

5. D

6. D

7. C

8. C

9. A

10. A

Exercise 2

1. The cranium consists of eight bones: frontal, occipital, right and left parietal, right and left temporal, sphenoid, and ethmoid.

2. The temporal bones contain the auditory canals. They are located in the petrous portion.

3. The orbits are made up of the frontal bone, ethmoid bone, lacrimal bones, maxilla, and zygoma.

4. The bones that contain paranasal sinuses are the maxilla, the ethmoid bone, the sphenoid bone, and the frontal bone.

5. The cranial base is best demonstrated using the submentovertical (SMV) projection.

6. For both projections, the sagittal plane of the skull and the orbitomeatal line are perpendicular to the film. In both projections, the central ray is angled 30 degrees. For the AP axial (Towne) projection, the central ray is angled caudad and for the PA axial (reverse Towne) projection it is angled cephalad.

7. The Waters and lateral projections.

8. The lateral projection of the nasal bones is done tabletop (non-Bucky) using detail screens, and the lateral projection of the facial bones is done using the Bucky with rapid screens. The radiation field is smaller for the nasal bones than for the lateral projection of the facial bones.

9. The patient is prone or seated, facing the Bucky with the chin resting on the table or the upright Bucky with the neck extended so that the orbitomeatal line forms an angle of 37 degrees with the film. The central ray is perpendicular to the film through the acanthion.

10. When the petrous ridge is projected over the floor of the maxillary sinuses, more extension of the neck is necessary. Further extension of the neck will project the petrous ridge below the maxillary sinuses.

11. Blow-out fracture: parietoacanthial (Waters) projection
Nasal bone fracture: lateral projection of nasal bones
Zygomatic arch fracture: submentovertical (SMV) or verticosubmental (VSM) projection
Mandible fracture(s): PA and oblique semiaxial projections

12. Multiple myeloma
Osteoma
Pituitary adenoma
Paget disease

Exercise 3

Fig. 19-1
1. Frontal bone
2. Supraorbital foramen

3. Optic foramen
4. Superior orbital fissure
5. Temporal bone
6. Sphenoid bone
7. Parietal bone
8. Glabella
9. Bregma
10. Coronal suture
11. Squamosal suture
12. Lambda
13. Lambdoidal suture
14. Occipital bone
15. External occipital protuberance (inion)
16. Asterion
17. External acoustic meatus
18. Mastoid process
19. Styloid process
20. Glabella
21. Sphenoid bone
22. Pterion
23. Frontal bone
24. Parietal bone
25. Squamous portion of temporal bone
26. Occipital bone
27. Internal acoustic meatus
28. Petrous portion of temporal bone
29. Clivus
30. Pterygoid hamulus
31. Sphenoidal sinus
32. Ethmoid bone
33. Crista galli
34. Frontal sinus
35. Frontal bone
36. Crista galli
37. Cribriform plate
38. Optic canal and foramen
39. Tuberculum sellae
40. Anterior clinoid process
41. Sella turcica
42. Posterior clinoid process
43. Foramen lacerum
44. Dorsum sellae
45. Jugular foramen
46. Hypoglossal canal
47. Foramen magnum
48. Occipital bone
49. Clivus (dashed line)
50. Petrous portion
51. Diploe
52. Temporal bone
53. Foramen spinosum
54. Foramen ovale
55. Optic groove
56. Greater wing
57. Lesser wing
58. Orbital plate
59. Anterior

60. Middle
61. Posterior

Fig. 19-2

1. Optic groove
2. Optic canal
3. Greater wing
4. Foramen ovale
5. Foramen spinosum
6. Carotid sulcus
7. Dorsum sellae
8. Sella turcica
9. Posterior clinoid process
10. Tuberculum sellae
11. Foramen rotundum
12. Anterior clinoid process
13. Lesser wing
14. Superior orbital fissure
15. Greater wing
16. Medial pterygoid lamina
17. Lateral pterygoid lamina
18. Pterygoid hamulus
19. Sella turcica (contains pituitary gland)
20. Dorsum sellae
21. Posterior clinoid process
22. Anterior clinoid process

Fig. 19-3

1. Squamous portion
2. Zygomatic process
3. Articular tubercle
4. Mandibular fossa
5. Styloid process
6. Tympanic portion
7. Mastoid process
8. Mastoid portion
9. External acoustic meatus
10. Mastoid antrum
11. Arcuate eminence
12. Semicircular canal
13. Petrous ridge
14. Petrous apex
15. Carotid canal
16. Promontory (formed by cochlear base)
17. Mastoid process
18. Mastoid air cells
19. Squamous portion

Fig. 19-4

1. Nasal bone
2. Lacrimal bone
3. Optic foramen
4. Ethmoid bone
5. Infraorbital foramen
6. Inferior nasal concha
7. Anterior nasal spine (acanthion)

8. Mental protuberance
9. Mandible
10. Maxilla
11. Vomer
12. Temporal process
13. Zygoma
14. Inferior orbital fissure
15. Superior orbital fissure
16. External acoustic meatus
17. Mandibular condyle
18. Angle (gonion)
19. Mandibular notch
20. Coronoid process
21. Mandible
22. Mental foramen
23. Maxilla
24. Alveolar process
25. Zygoma
26. Anterior nasal spine (acanthion)
27. Nasal bone
28. Lacrimal bone
29. Ethmoid bone
30. Zygomatic arch
31. Clivus
32. Pterygoid hamulus
33. Palatine bone
34. Maxilla
35. Vomer
36. Ethmoid bone
37. Nasal bone
38. Crista galli
39. Frontal sinus
40. Frontal bone

Fig. 19-5

1. Ethmoid sinuses
2. Sphenoid sinuses
3. Maxillary sinuses
4. Intersinus septum
5. Frontal sinuses
6. Frontal sinus
7. Maxillary sinus
8. Sphenoid sinus
9. Ethmoid air cells
10. Posterior
11. Middle
12. Anterior

Fig. 19-6

1. Crista galli
2. Inferior orbital margin
3. Ethmoid sinus
4. Petrous ridge
5. Superior orbital margin
6. Dorsum sellae
7. Frontal sinus

Fig. 19-7
1. Inferior orbital margin
2. Petrous ridge
3. Ethmoid sinus
4. Superior orbital fissure
5. Superior orbital margin
6. Crista galli
7. Frontal sinus

Fig. 19-8
1. Parietal bone
2. Occipital bone
3. Petrous portion of temporal bone
4. Foramen magnum

Fig. 19-9
1. Parietal bone
2. Occipital bone
3. Mastoid portion of temporal bone
4. Acoustic meatuses
5. Sella turcica
6. Sphenoid wings
7. Frontal bone

Fig. 19-10
1. Petrous portion of temporal bone
2. Orbit
3. Frontal bone
4. Parietal bone

Fig. 19-11
1. Frontal bone
2. Superior orbital rim
3. Petrous ridge
4. Nasal septum

Fig. 19-12
1. Orbit
2. Zygoma
3. Maxillary sinus
4. Petrous ridge
5. Nasal septum
6. Inferior orbital rim

Fig. 19-13
1. Superimposed sphenoid wings
2. Lateral orbital rim
3. Maxilla
4. Mandible

Fig. 19-14
1. Zygomatic arch
2. Temporal process of zygomatic bone

Fig. 19-15
1. Orbit
2. Maxillary sinus
3. Petrous ridge
4. Sphenoid sinus
5. Nasal septum

Fig. 19-16
1. Frontal sinus
2. Ethmoid sinuses
3. Maxillary sinuses
4. Sphenoid sinus

Fig. 19-17
1. Sphenoid sinuses
2. Mandible
3. Ethmoid sinuses

Chapter 20

1. Geriatrics

2. Pediatrics

3. Wrap the infant snugly.
   Hold the infant gently but firmly; provide gentle motion.
   Hold the infant where the infant can see your face.
   Talk or sing to the infant softly while you work.

4. True

5. Show disapproval by not smiling and using a calm, firm tone to give instructions.
   Praise any attempt to show the right response.

6. A valid choice is one in which both possibilities are acceptable.

7. False

8. True

9. False

10. To prevent motion blur on the image from movement of the patient's arms and legs

11. Clavicles, hips

12. Ossification is incomplete.
    The head is larger in proportion to body size.
    The spine has a single, C-shaped curvature rather than multiple curves.

Muscle and bone tissues are less dense.
The subcutaneous fat layer is thicker before age 4.

13. True

14. 13 cm - 8 cm = 5 cm (difference in size)
5 cm × 2 kVp = 10 kVp (kVp change)
70 - 10 = 60 kVp
5 mAs × 0.8 (80%) = 4 mAs
New technique for the child would be 4 mAs at
60 kVp, 40 inches SID, nongrid.

15. High. A high mA setting permits the use of shorter
exposure times, which helps prevent motion blur on
the image.

16. To demonstrate failure of a lung segment to expand.
This helps to identify the location of a bronchial
blockage, even when an aspirated object cannot be
seen on a radiograph.

17. Greenstick

18. Wrist

19. Battered child syndrome or physical child abuse

20. All of the following are possible answers to this
question:
Multiple injuries
Evidence of chronic or repeated injury with no other
explanation
Injuries that are not consistent with the parents'
report of the trauma
Failure to seek prompt treatment for serious injury
Bruise marks shaped like hands, fingers, or objects
(such as a belt)
Specific patterns of scalding (seen when a conscious
child is immersed in hot water)
Burns from an electric stove, radiator, heater, or
other hot objects on the child's hands or buttocks
Cigarette burns on exposed areas or the genitals
Black eyes in an infant
Human bite marks
Lash marks
Choke marks around neck
Circular marks around wrists or ankles (twisting)
Separated skull sutures or bulging fontanel
Unexplained unconsciousness in an infant

21. Increasing

22. All of the following are possible answers to this
question:
Have their attention before you begin to speak.

Face the person, preferably with light on your face.
Lip reading may be an important supplement to
their hearing.
Hearing loss is frequently in the upper register, so
speak lower and louder. Do not shout.
Speak clearly at a moderate pace.
Avoid noisy background situations.
Rephrase when you are not understood.
Avoid potential misunderstandings by asking open-
ended questions.
Validate understanding by asking patients to repeat
instructions.
Be patient.

23. Organic brain syndrome

24. Recent events

25. Loss of calcium content in the bones

26. Muscle atrophy

Loss of subcutaneous fat

Loss of skin elasticity

Vein fragility (tendency to bruise)

27. Decubitus ulcers

28. Decrease, kVp

29. Diverticulitis

30. Parkinson disease

Chapter 21

Exercise 1

1. D

2. C

3. B

4. A

5. D

6. C

7. False

8. True

9. D

10. False

11. True

12. D

13. C

14. B

15. A

16. A

17. C

18. B

Exercise 2

1. I AM ExPERT

2. I   Identification (clear and complete, matches requisition)
   A Anatomy (necessary anatomy included and visible)
   M Marking (right or left)
   Ex Exposure (appropriate exposure factors used)
   P   Processing (any evidence of darkroom fog or handling artifacts)
   E   Esthetic considerations (artistic merit)
   R Radiation safety (evidence of collimation and shielding)
   T Troubleshooting (identification of problems and how to improve if repeat radiograph is necessary)

3. The anatomic position is the position in which the patient is standing erect, with the face directed forward, arms extended by the sides with the palms facing forward, and the toes pointing anteriorly.

4. View box bulbs should be changed every 2 years, even if they are working. This ensures that optimal light is always available to view images

Chapter 22

1. Application of specialized knowledge in a way that benefits others
   A high degree of responsibility to the community the profession serves
   Organization by the profession to govern itself
   Standards of professional behavior, education, and qualification to practice

  Enforcement of standards within the profession
  Publication of a peer-reviewed journal

2. False

3. True

4. Morals: right actions based on religious teachings. *Example:* It is wrong to steal (lie, murder, cheat, etc.).
   Values: the priority that is placed on the significance of various moral concepts. *Example:* "Right to life" and "right to choose" are both widely held values with respect to termination of pregnancy.
   Ethics: rules that apply values and moral standards to actions. *Example:* It is wrong to gossip (be disloyal, betray a confidence, threaten another, etc.).

5. American Registry of Radiologic Technologists (ARRT) Code of Ethics

6. ARRT Rules of Ethics

7. Principle 1: behaves professionally; responds to patient needs; supports colleagues; provides quality patient care
   Principle 2: shows respect for human dignity
   Principle 3: does not discriminate
   Principle 4: practices appropriately
   Principle 5: uses careful, responsible judgment
   Principle 6: provides information to physicians; does not diagnose or interpret images
   Principle 7: meets accepted standards of practice; minimizes radiation exposure
   Principle 8: practices ethical conduct; protects the patient's right to quality care
   Principle 9: respects confidentiality
   Principle 10: participates in professional activities and continuing education

8. True

9. False

10. Identify the problem.
    Develop alternate solutions.
    Select the best solution.
    Defend your selection.

11. Rights nos. 1, 5, 6, and 10.

12. False

13. False

14. True

15. Practicing outside the legal requirements may result in fines, loss of credentials, or even imprisonment. Failure to maintain the qualifications required by your employer may result in termination of your employment. Infractions of laws or professional rules may make it impossible for you to obtain professional standing and/or employment as a radiographer in the future.

16. 1. F

    2. B

    3. A

    4. D

    5. C

    6. G

17. Negligence

18. The doctrine of the reasonably prudent person

19. HIPAA

20. Malpractice

21. *Respondeat superior*

22. Identify patients properly
    Administer medications accurately
    Comply with all patient safety requirements
    Chart information correctly

23. Love and acceptance: 3
    Nutrition and oxygen: 1
    Recognition: 5
    Recreation: 4
    Self-actualization: 6
    Safety: 2

24. Any of the following are acceptable answers to this question:
    Stay home and care for yourself when ill or under severe psychologic stress.
    Ensure proper nutrition.
    Get regular exercise.
    Develop good sleep habits.
    Use good body mechanics when lifting and moving heavy objects.
    Follow infection control precautions, including getting hepatitis B vaccination.
    Follow radiation safety precautions.

25. Be a good listener.
    Use praise and appreciation as positive reinforcements when work is well done or when others go out of their way to offer assistance.
    Demonstrate respect for your co-workers as individuals by avoiding cliques and gossip.

26. Empathy

27. Focus on the needs of the patient.

28. To stay abreast of current trends and technology
    To maintain interest in work
    To learn new skills and expand knowledge
    To qualify for a promotion or a new position
    To meet colleagues and share information with them

29. A smile or pleasant facial expression
    Open posture, leaning forward toward another
    Positive touch

30. The listener confirmed understanding of the message.

31. Be nonjudgmental in both verbal and nonverbal communication.
    Do not allow the inappropriate actions or speech of an upset individual to goad you into a similar response.
    When you are uncertain whether the listener has understood you, request an answer.

32. Examples from the text: "Would you like a blanket over your knees?" and "Would you like to stop in the restroom before we begin?"

33. 1. D

    2. E

    3. A

    4. C

    5. B

34. Does not respond to noises or words spoken out of the range of vision
    Uses lip movements without making a sound or speaks in a flat monotone
    Points to the ears and mouth while shaking the head in a negative motion
    Uses gestures or writing motions to express the need for paper and pencil

35. American Sign Language (ASL)
    Lip reading and speech
    Reading and writing

36. False

37. False

38. True

39. Eye contact, interpersonal distance, gestures, and speed and tone of speech

40. It brings bad luck to compliment a child without also touching the child.

41. The United States, Hispanic culture, Russian culture

42. Fear or anxiety

43. Direct them to a comfortable waiting area; show interest and concern; provide practical information such as the length of the procedure and the destination of the patient afterward; and direct them to services, such as restrooms and telephones.

44. Chart

45. The institution in which they are produced

46. Obtain patient's signed consent; record the date, name and address of the physician requesting the images; send only those images requested; send images by mail or courier, if time permits.

Chapter 23

1. Fuel, oxygen, heat

2. False

3. True

4. No smoking
   No open flames
   No use of ungrounded appliances

5. The main evacuation route from your area and at least one alternate route
   A general layout of your facility's floor plan
   The locations of fire extinguishers and fire alarms
   The procedure for reporting a fire

6. RACE
   Rescue
   Alarm
   Contain
   Evacuate/extinguish

7. P: Pull the pin.
   A: Aim the nozzle.
   S: Squeeze the handle.
   S: Sweep. Use a sweeping motion from side to side.

8. Water

9. Limit access to the area.
   Evaluate the risks involved.
   Obtain both the information and the equipment to clean up the spill safely.
   Clean up the spill.
   If you lack the necessary skill or equipment, call your supervisor.

10. Body mechanics

11. Bend at the hips and knees

12. Push it

13. A. Fowler
    B. Sims
    C. Trendelenburg
    D. Knee-chest
    E. Lithotomy

14. Knees

15. Orthopnea

16. Fowler, lateral recumbent

17. Decubitus ulcers

18. Under the shoulders; under the knees

19. Lateral recumbent

20. Orthostatic hypotension

21. Weak side

22. The patient backs into the wheelchair to sit down

23. True

24. True

25. False. An incident report should be completed for any event that results in injury or potential harm.

26. Infectious organism
    Reservoir of infection
    Susceptible host
    Means of transmission

27. 1. F

    2. D

    3. G

    4. B

    5. C

    6. H

    7. A

    8. E

28. 1. Fomite: an object that has been in contact with pathogenic organisms; examples in the radiology department might include the x-ray table, upright Bucky, cassettes, calipers, and positioning sponges that are contaminated with infectious body fluids.
    2. Vector: an arthropod (insect, spider, or similar form) in whose body an infectious organism develops or multiplies before becoming infective to a new host; examples include the mosquito that spreads malaria and the tick that spreads Lyme disease.
    3. Vehicle: any medium that transports microorganisms; examples include contaminated food, water, drugs, and blood.
    4. Airborne contamination: contact with dust containing either endospores or droplet nuclei; examples include the droplet nuclei that spread tuberculosis and chickenpox.
    5. Droplet contamination: contact of the mucous membranes of the eyes, nose, or mouth of a susceptible person with droplets containing microorganisms; examples include droplets of mucus that might be spread through coughing or sneezing, spreading colds and flu.

29. The Centers for Disease Control and Prevention (CDC)

30. Human immunodeficiency virus (HIV)

31. Sexual intercourse, sharing contaminated needles

32. True

33. True

34. False

35. Blood, blood products, or body fluids

36. A and E

37. Hepatitis B virus (HBV)

38. Within 2 hours of the exposure

39. Airborne droplet nuclei that are generated when an infected person coughs or speaks (the airborne contamination route)

40. False

41. True

42. Tuberculin skin test, also called Mantoux test or purified protein derivative (PPD) test

43. Blood
    All body fluids and wound drainage
    Secretions and excretions (except sweat), regardless of whether they contain visible blood
    Mucous membranes

44. Methicillin-resistant *Staphylococcus aureus* (MRSA)
    vancomycin-resistant enterococci (VRE)
    Penicillin-resistant *Streptococcus*
    Pseudomonas aeruginosa
    Clostridium difficile

45. Disinfection

46. Surgical asepsis or sterilization

47. Hand hygiene

48. True

49. False

50. When hands are visibly soiled or contaminated with blood or body fluid or when contamination by endospores is suspected

51. A diluted solution of sodium hypochlorite bleach (Clorox)

52. Biohazard

53. True

54. False. Recapping is a common cause of needle sticks.

55. Sharps container

56. Autoclaving or steam sterilization

57. Gas sterilization

58. Sterile field

59. They are clean, dry, and unopened.
    Their expiration date has not been exceeded.
    Their sterility indicators have changed to a predetermined color, confirming sterilization.

60. Away from you

61. False

62. True

63. True

64. Application

Chapter 24

1. Observation, evaluation, and assessment

2. Touch patients reassuringly and tell them what to expect.
   Respect patient's modesty.
   Let them know when you leave the area and when you expect to return.
   Escort ambulatory patients to and from various areas of the facility.

3. If the patient feels chilled, provide a blanket.
   Provide a drink of water if appropriate.
   Be sensitive to the need for elimination and assist as needed.

4. Incontinence

5. Onset
   Duration
   Specific location
   Quality of pain
   What aggravates
   What alleviates

6. Cyanotic

7. Perspiring

8. A fever

9. Higher

10. Lower

11. When the patient has recently had a hot or cold beverage, is receiving oxygen, or breathes through the mouth

12. Tachycardia

13. Weak and rapid

14. Systolic

15. High

16. B

17. Never borrow equipment or supplies from the emergency set for routine use.
    When you use these items in an emergency, be sure that supplies are replenished and the kit is ready for use before returning it to storage.

18. Mask

19. 3 to 5 L/min

20. Less

21. Suction

22. A heart attack

23. Initiate the "shake and shout" maneuver

24. Irreparable brain damage

25. Fibrillation

26. Intracranial pressure

27. Contrecoup injury

28. Alert and conscious
    Drowsy but responsive
    Unconscious but reactive to painful stimuli
    Comatose

29. Compound fracture

30. Hemorrhage

31. Erythema

32. Anaphylaxis or anaphylactic shock

33. A moderate allergic response, such as urticaria

34. An allergic reaction

35. Diabetic coma

36. Insulin

37. Stroke

38. Slurred or difficult speech
    Extreme dizziness
    Severe headache
    Muscle weakness on one or both sides
    Difficulty in vision or deviation in one eye
    Temporary loss of consciousness

39. Stroke

40. Keep the patient as safe as possible

41. Seizure

42. Try to persuade the patient to breathe more slowly
    or to breathe into a paper bag.

43. Fainting

44. Vertigo

45. Epistaxis

Chapter 25

1. Checking the allergy history of the patient
   Preparing medication for administration
   Verifying patient identification
   Assisting the physician
   Monitoring the patient after the medication has
   been given

2. It is the physician's duty

3. True

4. False

5. Generic name

6. Proprietary or trade name

7. 1. D
   2. A
   3. E
   4. C
   5. B

8. The U.S. Food and Drug Administration (FDA)

9. Effectiveness

10. Strength

11. 1. H
    2. C
    3. F
    4. E
    5. A
    6. B
    7. D
    8. G

12. 1. E
    2. A
    3. D
    4. A
    5. B
    6. D
    7. C

13. Hydration

14. 1. C
    2. B
    3. A
    4. D

15. Receptor sites on cells

16. Therapeutic effect

17. Controlled

18. Opiates, opioids, and benzodiazepines

19. An antidote

20. 40 lb × 0.45 = 18 kg

21. 3 ml

22. 150 mcg

23. True

24. False

25. Vastus lateralis muscle of the thigh

26. 18 to 20

27. The intravenous solution has infiltrated.

28. Shut off the flow of fluid, notify a nurse or physician, remove the needle or catheter from the vein, and apply cold packs to the affected area.

29. True

30. True

31. Date and time, name of drug, dose, route of administration, identification of person charting

Chapter 26

1. All pathogens, principally human immunodeficiency virus, hepatitis B virus, and hepatitis C virus

2. All patients' body fluids are potentially infectious.

3. Hand hygiene
   Barrier techniques
   Proper disposal of contaminated waste

4. Biohazardous waste

5. Sharps container

6. Venipuncture

7. Antecubital fossa (front side of the elbow)

8. The presence or absence of specific additives

9. Tubes with additives should be filled after those that have no additives.
   Tubes with additives must be gently inverted after filling to ensure adequate mixing.

10. True

11. 21 gauge; 1 or 1½ inches

12. The stopper of the evacuated collection tube; the skin

13. True

14. False

15. Tourniquet

16. Blood cultures; blood alcohol testing

17. False. Shielding is necessary for safety, even with these special tubes.

18. Above the site where intravenous fluids are being infused
    Where excess scarring is evident
    The arm on the side of a mastectomy

19. Palpation

20. After

21. Before

22. The needle is not properly situated in the lumen (channel) of the vein.

23. Urinalysis

24. Macroscopic examination of physical characteristics
    Chemical analysis performed with a urine reagent strip
    Microscopic examination of the urine sediment

25. Recap the bottle immediately after a strip is removed and store the bottle at room temperature.

26. False

27. When the patient awakens in the morning; this is called a *first morning specimen.*

28. Random specimen

29. Clean-catch midstream specimen (CCMS) technique

30. Anterior to posterior

31. The specimen should be capped, protected from light, and refrigerated until the analysis is performed; before analysis, it should be warmed to room temperature, gently remixed, and transferred to a urinalysis tube.

32. Color
    Appearance (clarity)

33. True

34. The specimen should be sent to a laboratory for analysis by a different method.

35. "Positive for nonhemolyzed blood"

36. The CCMS technique is employed immediately after the insertion of a fresh tampon.

37. Hazy urine (more than slightly hazy); positive results for glucose, protein, blood, nitrite, or leukocyte esterase

38. Centrifuge

Chapter 27

1. The weights on both calibration bars should be set at 0 and the scale should be in balance.

2. Lower

3. The patient's weight is determined by noting the readings on both calibration bars and adding them together.

4. The patient is not standing still.

5. Before

6. Quarter pound

7. Quarter inch

8. Myopia: nearsightedness
   Hyperopia: farsightedness
   Presbyopia: farsightedness associated with advancing age

9. Snellen E

10. 20 feet

11. Right eye: OD

    Left eye: OS

12. Ishihara

13. Electrocardiogram

14. 1. P wave

    2. P-R segment

    3. S-T segment

    4. T wave

    5. U wave

    6. P-R interval

    7. Q wave

    8. QRS complex

    9. S wave

    10. Q-T interval

15. Standard leads (limb or bipolar leads): I, II and III
    Augmented leads: aVR, aVL, and aVF
    Precordial (chest) leads: V_1, V_2, V_3, V_4, V_5, and V_6

16. Wave amplitude

17. Record the ECG at the ½ STD setting

18. 25 mm/sec

19. Must be connected to a specific electrode

20. 1. D

    2. B

    3. G

    4. E

    5. A

    6. F

    7. C

21. Electrolyte

22. True

23. An exercise tolerance test or an ECG stress test

24. Spirometry

25. Volume-displacement type
    Flow-sensing type

26. Flow-volume spirogram
    Time-volume spirogram

27. An immediate forceful start
    A maximum effort
    A smooth continuous exhalation that does not end abruptly

28. Three

29. Eight (After eight attempts, fatigue prevents accurate testing.)

30. Recent abdominal surgery
    Recent thoracic surgery
    Recent eye surgery, including cataract operations
    Hemoptysis (coughing up blood) from an unknown cause
    Pneumothorax (collapsed lung)

Chapter 28

Exercise 1

1. C

2. D

3. D

4. A

5. A

6. B

7. B

8. B

9. B

10. D

Exercise 2

1. Old bone is replaced with new bone. Osteoclast are the bone-destroying cells. Osteoblasts are the bone-building cells.

2. Beneath the table and the patient

3. Eliminate the contribution of soft tissue and measure the attenuation due to bone alone. Scan at two different x-ray photon energies and mathematically manipulate the recorded signal. The density of the isolated bone is calculated on the principle that denser, more mineralized bone produces more x-ray attenuation.

4. Pencil beam, fan array, and cone beam

5. BMD = BMC/Area

6. Pregnancy, recent barium or other contrast media studies

7. Accuracy is equipment dependent and relates to the ability to measure the true BMD. Precision is technologist related and involves the ability to reproduce positioning.

8. Time
   Distance
   Shielding

9. 1 m for pencil beam and 3 m for fan array

10. Primary: osteoporosis related to postmenopausal status (type I), or aging (type II)
    Secondary: osteoporosis caused by other factors, such as medications or disease processes

11. Lumbar spine and proximal femur

12. Repeat the test and record the problem or corrective action.
    If the tests fails a second time, call the manufacturer's help or applications service line.
    Cancel all patient appointments until the problem is resolved.

Exercise 3

Match the following terms with their definitions.

1. H
2. U
3. V
4. M
5. B
6. D
7. E
8. L
9. N
10. F
11. A
12. S
13. O
14. P
15. Y
16. W
17. J
18. C
19. I
20. K
21. X
22. Q
23. G
24. R
25. T

Exercise 4

1. Yes. There are six lumbar vertebrae. Based on the densitometric shape the labeling is correct. It is important for technologists to understand densitometric anatomy and the shape of the individual vertebral bodies. It is imperative to acquire and analyze consistently when obtaining serial scans

2. A. Compression fracture is seen at L1. The compression fracture at L1 will falsely increase the BMD if results for L1 through L4 are reported.

   B. Reanalyze excluding L1 and/or just report on L2 through L4 for a comparison of equal area.

3. Greater trochanter: 4
   Femoral neck: 6
   Femoral head: 5
   Pelvic ischium: 3
   Lesser trochanter: 1
   Femoral shaft: 2

4. Compression fracture has occurred at L1.
   The image shows a smaller, more compact area, and increased density or brighter image.

5. Ulna: 4
   Radius: 2
   Distal radius: 1
   Proximal ulna: 3
   Ulnar styloid: 5